PDNT Book 2
Cancer nursing

PROFESSIONAL
Development

NURSING TIMES NT

Published by
Emap Healthcare, part of Emap Business Communications Ltd
Porters South
4 Crinan Street
London N1 9XW

Companies and representatives throughout the world
Film output (repro) by David Bruce Graphics
Printed in Great Britain by Drogher Press, Christchurch, Dorset

ISBN 1 902499 00 X

Contents

CONTRIBUTORS

Art editor: Amanda Davies
Coordinator: Fiona Lane
Editor: Rob Garbett
Illustration: Peter Gardiner
Marketing: Sophie Wybrew-Bond
Production: Andrew Sumner
Publisher: John Barnes
Sub-editor: Julia Bell

Breast cancer:
Author: Barbara Chaplin, RGN, Macmillan breast care nurse, Grimsby Health NHS Trust

Digestive tract cancers:
Authors: Teresa Finlay, BSc, RGN, senior nurse, practice development, University Hospital Birmingham NHS Trust; Sarah Burns, BA, RGN, SCM, DipN ed, professional development adviser

Leukaemia:
Authors: Ken Campbell, FIBMS, SRMLSO, MIHSM, CertHMS, information officer, Leukaemia Research Fund; Tim Jackson, SRN, RM, RNMS, lead nurse, haematology directorate, University College Hospital

Palliative care:
Author: Chris Bailey, MSc, BA, RGN, project coordinator, Institute of Cancer Research; Julia Downing, BN, DipCN, RGN, is lecturer in cancer nursing, Institute of Cancer Nursing; Shaun Kinghorn, BA, RGN, RNT, RCNT, lecturer in cancer and palliative care studies, Marie Curie Centre

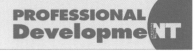

CONTENTS

Keep yourself up to date

Use your reading as a vital part of your professional updating

Welcome to *Nursing Times'* Professional Development Book 2. It follows on from our popular Professional Development *Nursing Times* series (PDNT), which ran for over three years.

The contents have been revised and updated to ensure that they reflect contemporary thinking in the areas concerned. The books are designed for busy clinical nurses looking to update their knowledge and skills, for students and for practitioners returning to work after a break.

Each unit concludes with a multiple choice questionnaire for you to test your knowledge. This book and others in the series provide you with one means to keep up to date and relate your learning practice so that you can meet the UKCC's standards for post registration education (PREP).

This book uses *Nursing Times* Study Hours to help you keep a record of what you learn and how long it took you.

PROFESSIONAL DevelopmeNT

PREP MADE SIMPLE

Lifelong learning is an important part of every nurse's working life. The UKCC has provided a framework to help nurses relate their learning to practice in order to provide safe and effective practice.

While there has been a degree of anxiety about how to meet the minimum requirement of five days study or its equivalent, we at *Nursing Times* believe that reading the professional press can be of great help.

Study Hours have been designed by *Nursing Times* to provide an easy-to-use estimation of the time you spend reflecting on and studying clinical issues. Using Study Hours puts you in control of your own professional development and helps you meet the PREP requirements.

THE STUDY HOURS RATING

The Study Hours rating is the figure inside the clock. It is our estimate of the number of hours it will take you to read and reflect on the material provided.

The figure given is our estimate but it does not matter if you take more or less time; record the time you spend in your professional profile.

STUDY HOURS IN PRACTICE

Reading articles, supplements and publications such as this can be a passive affair but it can also, if you choose, be the starting point of a great deal of reflection and practice-related activity.

For example, imagine a nurse in a genito-urinary clinic reading something in *NT* about dying with dignity: an article looking at different cultural beliefs surrounding death. Although working with death is not usually a feature of her working day, the nurse realises that sexuality and sexual taboos are very significant in the location where she works, which has a large population from an Asian background.

The nurse realises that despite this, relatively few Asian clients present at her clinic so she investigates further to find out what social and cultural factors might be at work.

As a result of her research the nurse is able to establish an outreach network with local community centres, social clubs and places of work where she gives talks and hands out information in a number of languages stressing the need for early investigation and treatment of genito-urinary disease.

All this activity represents activity relevant to meeting PREP requirements and comes from reading the professional press. We hope that the materials in the book will similarly stimulate your personal and professional development.

Breast cancer
Knowledge for practice

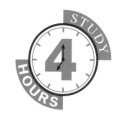

Breast cancer is the most common form of cancer among women in the UK and is also the most common cause of all deaths in women aged 35–44 years. The UK has the highest breast cancer mortality rate in the world although there has been a small but significant reduction over the past five years.[1] The highest incidence is seen in women over the age of 60. Over 31 000 new cases were diagnosed in 1989 in the UK and it is estimated that 15 000 women die of the disease each year.[1] One woman in 12 will develop breast cancer at some time. Male breast cancer is estimated at one in 200.

While the incidence of breast cancer varies widely from country to country, the highest rates are found in the most developed ones. However, there is an overall global rise in incidence: 26% more cases were recorded around the world in 1985 than in 1980.[2] It is now the most common form of cancer in women in North Africa, the Caribbean, west Asia, South America and Polynesia.

THE NORMAL BREAST

At birth both males and females have undeveloped breasts with small underdeveloped nipples. Breast development starts at puberty and is usually complete by 16–18 (Fig 1). The biological role of the breasts is to produce milk to nourish a baby.

The adult breast is roughly conical with a base that extends from the second to the sixth ribs from the sternal edge to the axillary line. Breast tissue also projects into the lower axilla and extends along the lower border of the pectoralis major. Slightly below the centre of each breast is a ring of pigmented skin known as the areola, which surrounds the central projecting nipple.

The inside of the breast consists of 15–20 lobes. In each lobe there are several smaller compartments called lobules. These are grape-like clusters composed of connective tissue in which milk-secreting alveoli glands are embedded. The alveoli glands drain into the lactiferous ducts. Nearer to the nipple the lactiferous sinuses act as a reservoir for potential milk. In the non-pregnant woman these are normally plugged with keratin. The lactiferous ducts end at the nipple where there are 10–15 openings that can deliver milk.

The lobes of the breast are separated by adipose and connective tissue. Breast size is largely dependent on the amount of adipose tissue deposited. The strands of connective tissue are called suspensory ligaments. These ligaments run between the skin and deep fascia and support the breast rather like a bra. Breasts lose their firmness because of loss of elasticity in these ligaments during lactation and ageing.

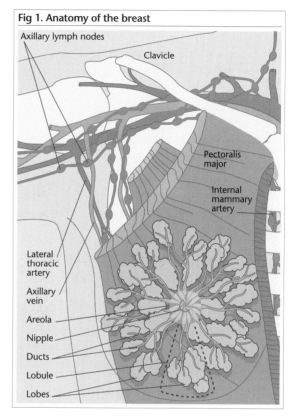

Fig 1. Anatomy of the breast

Axillary lymph nodes
Clavicle
Pectoralis major
Internal mammary artery
Lateral thoracic artery
Axillary vein
Areola
Nipple
Ducts
Lobule
Lobes

Lymph, blood and nervous supply
The lymph system rids the breast of waste products. The lymph vessels originate in a plexus in the interlobular spaces and in the walls of the lactiferous ducts. The efferent lymph vessels from the greater part of the breast join with the lymphatic plexus in the fascia of the pectoral muscle and end in the pectoral group of the axillary lymph nodes.

Major drainage is from the axilla and internal mammary chain. The axillary lymph nodes receive 75% of the lymph fluid from the breast; the remainder drains into the parasternal nodes.[2]

Blood is supplied from the perforating branches of the mammary artery, a relatively minor branch of the vessels coming off the aorta. Arterial supply is also derived from the thoracic branches of the axillary artery and from the internal thoracic and intercostal arteries. The venous drainage follows the arterial supply.

The sensory supply of the breast comes from the third to the sixth lateral intercostal nerves.

Table 1. Factors that affect risk for developing breast cancer

Factors that increase the risk of developing breast cancer are:

Age

Nulliparity

Late childbearing

Early menarche

Family history, especially first-degree relative

Obesity in post-menopausal women

Pre-menopausal exposure to ionising radiation

History of benign breast disease

Previous breast cancer

Hormone replacement therapy

Factors still under evaluation:

Alcohol intake

High-fat diet

Oral contraceptives use, especially prolonged use

Table 2. Staging of breast cancer

Once a cancer has been diagnosed, patients are staged using the TNM classification system, which classifies tumour size, lymph node involvement and metastatic spread

TIS	*In situ* breast cancer
T1	Tumour size below 2cm
T2	Above 2–5cm
T3	Above 5cm
T4a	Involvement of chest wall
T4b	Involvement of skin
T4c	T4a and T4b
T4d	Inflammatory cancer
N0	No regional node metastasis
N1	Mobile ipsilateral
N2	Fixed ipsilateral
N3	Internal mammary nodes involvement
M0	No evidence of metastasis
M1	Distant metastasis

Muscles

The principal muscles related to the breast are the pectoral major and pectoral minor, the serrator anterior and latissimus dorsi. The pectoral major is responsible for the contour of the chest wall and forms the front border of the axilla. To the left is the pectoral minor, a small muscle that arises from the third, fourth and fifth ribs and is inserted into the front of the shoulder blade. In the base of the armpit are two major muscles. The serator anterior arises from this and the side of the chest, and is inserted into the scapula, and the latissimus dorsi which originates from the back bone and is inserted in the humerus, forming the boundary at the back of the axilla.

Hormonal influence

Throughout the menstrual cycle the hormone oestrogen, stimulated by pituitary activity, flows to the breasts from the ovaries and the adrenal glands. It reaches its peak during the middle two weeks of the cycle. Cells multiply in the lobes and lobules of the breast as it comes under the influence of oestrogen in preparation for possible milk production and transport. Progesterone is released at mid-cycle. Blood supply increases to the breast to meet the additional needs of the working breast. If no pregnancy occurs, the extra fluid is returned to the body's general circulation via the lymph network in the breast.

During pregnancy placental oestrogen and progesterone levels are elevated. The alveoli develop and produce milk, which passes to the lactiferous ducts. In addition, the anterior pituitary gland in the brain releases the hormones prolactin. Breast size increases by approximately 45–50%.

Menopause

After the menopause most of the lobules become inactive and eventually there is a loss of glandular tissue, particularly in the lobules, as the monthly hormonal cycles decline and stop. There is also an increase of fat deposition. Fatty tissue, unlike glandular tissue, shows up clearly on X-ray. The increased hormonal activity in younger women makes mammography images appear cloudy. Routine mammogram screening begins at age 50.

In older age the breast mainly consists of fatty tissue with a few resident ducts. Externally these changes produce the shrunken pendulous breast of the older woman.

FAMILIAL BREAST CANCER

It has now been accepted that a strong family history, involving dominant genes contributes to about 5% of breast cancers (Table 1).[3] A woman with a first-degree relative (mother or sister) with breast cancer, particularly if the cancer was diagnosed at a young age (before 45), pre-menopausally, or if the cancer is in both breasts, is at an increased risk. Over the past three years there have been substantial advances in the identification of genes that predispose women to familial breast cancer.

There may actually be six or more genes causing familial breast cancer. The most important of these identified so far is BRCa1, which has been located on the long arm of chromosome number 17. It is estimated to occur in 45% of families where breast cancer is diagnosed under the age of 45. Possessing the gene carries an 80% risk of disease at the age of 80.

Fig 2. Breast changes associated with breast cancer

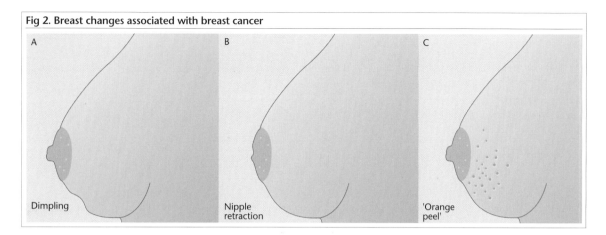

A — Dimpling
B — Nipple retraction
C — 'Orange peel'

Another gene is P53, which is the most commonly altered gene in human cancers. Germ-line mutations in this gene have been found in 50% of families with Li-fraumeni syndrome.[3] Gene carriers in Li-fraumeni families are identified as having a high risk of developing early-onset breast, ovarian and bowel cancer.

The genes located so far do not account for all cases of familial breast cancer. The knowledge about the mechanism of action of these genes will eventually direct new approaches to the treatment and prevention of the disease. The identification of carriers will enable targeted prevention of those at higher risk. Some genes may predispose to malignancies other than breast cancer, and this may alter the management of breast cancer.

Other risk factors
The risk of developing breast cancer increases with age. It is rare before the age of 25 years. However, the incidence increases just before menopause, following which there is a slight downward trend during the menopausal years, before the incidence rate rises again but at a slower rate with old age.[4]

For women who have an early onset of menarche (before the age of 12) there is a two to three times increase in the risk of breast cancer. Although age at menarche is an important factor, the time at which a woman establishes a regular ovulatory cycle may be more important. The relative risk occurring in young women who have regular ovulatory cycles before the age of 12 is nearly four times that of a woman whose menarche occurs after the age of 12 with regular ovulatory cycles starting after an interval of five years.

Oestrogens associated with hormonal activity have been extensively studied because of their important effects on the growth of the breast epithelium.[6]

Pregnancy
There is a decreased risk of breast cancer associated with pregnancy. The number of pregnancies a woman has is an important determinant of risk, but age at the time of the first full-term pregnancy has been shown in some studies, to be important.[4] A woman aged 20 when she has her first child has about half the risk of a woman who has not had a child. Women whose first full-term pregnancy occurs between the age of 30–34 years have approximately the same risk as that found in a nulliparous woman. Pregnancies after the age of 35 were associated with a slightly increased risk. Incomplete pregnancies before the first full term do not have any protective effect. An early age at the birth of the second child further reduces the risk of developing breast cancer.

A number of recent studies have found that three months or more of breast-feeding decreases the risk of breast cancer, particularly for premenopausal onset.[5]

Oral contraception and hormone replacement therapy
Epidemiological studies have found that oral contraceptive use does not affect the risk of breast cancer in the majority of women, regardless of dose, brand and type of oestrogen or progesterone. Some studies, however, have identified subgroups of oral contraceptive users who may have an increased risk; for example, women who have used oral contraception for several years before the age of 25 and/or before a first full-term pregnancy.[6]

The findings are by no means unanimous. Several studies have shown no association with oral contraceptive use in women over the age of 40. Recently there has been a suggestion of a slight reduction in risk with oral contraceptive use.[7] But there is also evidence from a national case study that a positive family history of breast cancer and prolonged oral contraceptive use increases risk.[8]

Studies concerned with whether there is an elevated risk of breast cancer among women who use hormone replacement therapy have produced conflicting results. Meta-analysis of worldwide studies of HRT and breast cancer suggest that it does increase the risk incrementally with length of use.[9] There is little data on the effects of combined oestrogen/progestogen used in the UK. Most

BREAST CANCER

studies relate to the use of oestrogen alone, and it may be some time before conclusive data for the UK becomes available. Menopause after the age of 55 doubles the risk of cancer developing.[4]

Other risk factors
There is direct evidence to suggest that exposure to ionising radiation, particularly between puberty and the age of 20 years when breast tissue is rapidly developing, can subsequently increase the risk of breast cancer.[4] Body weight and diet may also carry associated risks. Overweight postmenopausal women have both higher levels of androsterone to oestrogen in adipose tissue and lower levels of sex-hormone-binding globulin than do thinner women.

The risk of developing a second primary breast cancer is five times the general risk and is inversely related to age at presentation of the primary cancer: the younger the woman, the higher the risk of recurrence.[8]

TUMOUR GROWTH

The most common form of neoplasm occurring in the breast is infiltrating ductal carcinoma. It grows in the epithelial cells lining the ducts. Breast cancer is capable of rapid systemic spread. In its early stages it is non-invasive, affecting mainly the ducts. Once a lesion has reached 5mm in size it may invade the lymph nodes to enter the systemic circulation.

Tumours are most often situated in the upper outer quadrant of the breast. As it grows it becomes more attached to the chest wall or the overlying skin. Without treatment the surrounding tissues are invaded, extending to the lymph glands of the axilla. Metastasis occurs most often in the lungs, bones, mediastinal lymph nodes or liver. Without treatment death may occur in three years.

Clinical features
About 80% of symptomatic breast carcinomas appear as a palpable mass (Fig 2). A mobile lump appears, most frequently in the upper outer quadrant of the breast. There

may or may not be pain. If no lump is present, attention may be drawn to a problem by localised discomfort such as burning, stinging or aching. Less common presentation is nipple discharge and retraction. After a time, dimpling or 'orange peel' appearance of the skin may be observed. This is caused by shortening of the suspensory ligaments caused by fibrosis around the cancer. On examination, asymmetry and elevation of the breast may be observed. Advanced presentation include skin ulceration, skin nodules and skin oedema. Later, the breast becomes fixed to the chest wall and nodes are palpable in the axilla. Finally, ulceration occurs and general ill health and cathexia become evident.

Staging is used as a means of identifying the extent of disease progress to aid the judgement of appropriate treatment and likely prognosis.

Prognosis
Breast cancer is unpredictable because it is influenced by hormone levels, immune response, host resistance and other variable factors. Where lymph nodes have not been involved, prognosis is improved; however, the absence of nodes does not necessarily mean the absence of malignancy as growth may be microscopic. The extent of tumour spread at the time of treatment is more significant in prognosis (Table 2).

THINKING POINTS

● Breast-conserving surgery has not been as popular as originally predicted. Why might this be?
● When you encounter women with breast cancer, how aware are you of the individuals and organisations that can provide support with side-effects of the disease and treatment? Are there any areas of unmet need? How can this be addressed?

PART TWO

The role of the nurse

Many nurses care for women with breast cancer and their families. This can be in the community, in a hospital ward or in an out-patients' department. Nurses play an important role in the care that women receive, providing support in a time of frightening and sometimes unpleasant procedures and treatment for the disease.

Investigation brings with it uncertainty and fear, as well as the discomfort involved in the procedures themselves. Treatment, whether surgical or medical, causes discomfort, debility and change in body image. This is followed by the person with breast cancer having to cope with altered body image and the fear of recurrence or the knowledge of impending death.

INVESTIGATIONS FOR BREAST CANCER

Mammography is a soft tissue X-ray of the breast which can show changes that are not detectable on physical examination (Table 3). The breast is compressed between two plates while the exposure is made. This usually takes less than one minute and may feel uncomfortable. Mammography does not usually produce clear pictures in young women in their 20s and early 30s because their breast tissue is dense.

Ultrasound projects high-frequency sound waves into the breast. The sound waves bounce off tissue with different densities in distinct ways.

A computer reads the echo pattern, producing a visual representation of the breast. This method is useful for patients of all ages, as tissue density does not affect ability to interpret images.

Tissue samples can be gathered in a number of ways. Fine-needle aspiration cytology (FNCA) requires the insertion of a fine needle into a lesion. The aspirated breast cells are sent for cytology. Core biopsy involves the removal of a core sample of tissue from the lump, using a cutting needle.

The patient may be bruised and feel sore in the days following. Nipple cytology involves scraping cells from the nipple or obtaining a direct impression of the nipple on to a clean glass slide which is sent for cytological analysis.

The more invasive procedure of excision open biopsy may be required. An open biopsy aims to remove a palpable lesion with a minimal area of surrounding breast tissue.

It is performed under a general anaesthetic. The area to be excised may be identified by inserting a wire into the lesion under X-ray guidance. Ultrasound may also be used to locate the lesion before surgery. This procedure is often used when the lesion in the breast is impalpable.

Nursing care and investigations
Many women state that the time between finding the lump and having a diagnosis confirmed is the most stressful. Nurses who work in surgical out-patients departments and breast clinics are ideally placed to ensure that women are supported through this stressful time. An important factor is that bad news should be given in the most appropriate way, in a suitable setting.

Where possible patients should be encouraged to have someone with them when learning of their diagnosis. The presence of a close relative or friend during the breaking of bad news has been reported as reducing the incidence of anxiety and depression in patients monitored over 12 months.[10] The shock of learning a diagnosis often hinders the assimilation of information.

Not all patients tell their families about the discovery of a breast lump and may prefer to keep their fears to themselves and go through the investigations alone. They may try to protect those close to them.

There is evidence to suggest that the use of audiotapes helps patients psychologically. Audiotapes can help a patient to recall information about diagnosis, treatment

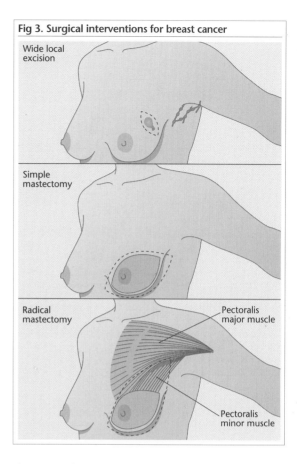

Fig 3. Surgical interventions for breast cancer

Wide local excision

Simple mastectomy

Radical mastectomy

Pectoralis major muscle

Pectoralis minor muscle

choices and further investigations, thus making it easier to share the bad news with the family, who may not be present at the consultation. The family plays an important role in the rehabilitation of the patient, and their support should be enlisted from early on.[11]

SURGICAL PROCEDURES

A range of surgical procedures is available in the treatment of breast cancer. Practice and beliefs vary from surgeon to surgeon as to the extent of surgery needed at different stages of the disease (Fig 3).
● Simple mastectomy involves removal of the breast tissue with overlying skin, usually including the nipple;
● Wide local excision of breast tissue involves the removal of cancer tissue with a margin of surrounding normal breast tissue;
● Subcutaneous mastectomy involves removing the internal breast tissue but leaving the nipple intact.

Axillary sampling or axillary clearance is usually done at the time of breast surgery. It involves removing a sample of the lymph glands or complete removal of all the axillary glands (Fig 4). Staging the extent of disease in the axilla is important for selecting the kind of subsequent therapy needed (Table 2).

Breast reconstruction

The reconstruction of the breast after mastectomy can take several forms. Tissue expansion is a procedure whereby a prosthesis is placed under the muscle and gradually expanded with saline over a number of weeks in order to stretch the overlying skin. This creates a pocket into which a synthetic implant can subsequently be placed.

Alternatively, a flap of skin, fat or muscle can be transferred from a donor site on the back or abdomen to the operative area. A new nipple may be created with tissue from the other nipple, the labia or thigh.

Breast reconstruction can be done immediately or can be delayed, depending on the patient's preference and the surgeon's advice.

Complications of surgery

Mastectomy wounds are prone to inflammatory and circulatory problems. Seroma can also occur in the dead space under the flap following mastectomy and can occur in wide excision surgery. It is caused by the transudation of fluid across the large internal surface area.

Infection, necrosis of the flap and lymphoedema of the arm on the side where the surgery took place can also occur. There is an increased risk of lymphoedema when both surgery and radiotherapy are performed on the axilla. Nurses are ideally placed in the surgical clinic to be aware of this development and to make appropriate referrals.

In the mid-1980s reports from randomised clinical trials comparing relapse-free intervals and survival in women with early breast cancer by mastectomy or wide local excision demonstrated no differences in survival between the two groups.[12]

As a result, some woman are encouraged during their surgical consultation to make a decision about surgical treatment. The majority of women appreciate the opportunity to be involved in the decision-making process. However, other women may feel overwhelmed and fearful of making the wrong decision. Nurses can play a valuable role in helping patients weigh up their choices. However, true respect for a patient's autonomy should include supporting the person's right to decline the offer to make her own decision.

The majority of patients appreciate clear information that explains the different policies. They may display information-seeking behaviour but it should not then be taken for granted that they want to shoulder the burden of decision-making.[13]

CARE AFTER SURGERY

Post-operative care is aimed at promoting freedom from pain and post-surgical complications. In the longer term, nurses are the primary source of support in helping patients come to terms with altered body image. They also support the patients with functional rehabilitation if the use of the arm is affected.

Pain relief is achieved through both analgesia and attention to position. Elevation of the arm affected by surgery will promote vascular and lymphatic drainage, and control swelling and pain. The patient may experience either numbness of the arm, or increased sensitivity.

Dressings and drains, when used, may also impede circulation, causing swelling and pain; these must be checked in the immediate postoperative period. The wound also must be closely observed for accumulation of fluid under the skin flap. This may be indicated by visible swelling. Wound drains should be checked for patency and the amount of drainage.

After surgery the patient should be encouraged to start exercising the arm as soon as possible. Early use of the arm promotes fluid return and prevents swelling. The fingers and the wrist can be exercised straight away, with gentle use of the whole arm being encouraged soon after. Shoulder stiffness and arm tightness is caused by fibrosis

---

Fig 4. Cervical, axillary and mammary lymph nodes

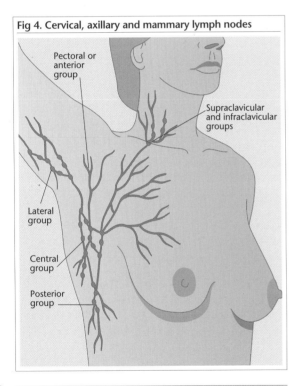

Pectoral or anterior group

Supraclavicular and infraclavicular groups

Lateral group

Central group

Posterior group

Table 3. Prediagnosis investigations for breast cancer

Specific to the breast	General
Mammogram	Full blood count
Ultrasound	Liver function test
Fine-needle aspiration	Chest X-ray
True-cut biopsy	Bone scan
Excision biopsy	Liver ultrasound

of the axillary suspensory ligaments. The nurse should work closely with the physiotherapist and give advice on activities involving use of the arm. More active exercises may be appropriate after the removal of sutures.

Infection is a risk, especially where there is a stagnant collection of blood products in the wound. Infection can delay healing and increase the risk of lymphoedema. It is important, therefore, to promote cleanliness and lack of irritation, which can be caused by creams or underarm deodorants used near the wound.

Altered body image

The nurse's role is important in observing and exploring the patient's feeling about the scar. The nurse may be the first person to react to the scar. Through touching the patient and the scar, the nurse can promote a feeling of normality. Even women who have had conservative surgery may feel that the cancer has violated their body; a small neat scar may still leave the patient with a profound sense of altered body image.[14]

To perform this role the nurse must have a certain degree of specialised knowledge. He or she must be aware of the concept of body image and be able to recognise the stages of adjustment a patient may go through, as well as coping methods. Support is particularly important when the patient first sees the area altered by surgery, particularly if there is distortion because of swelling or bruising. Care will also include dealing with the family's feelings.

Before a patient is discharged the nurse can offer to show her how to wear the temporary prosthesis. She may choose to wear this before discharge and experiment with her presentation to her family before she presents herself to the outside world.

The development of breast-conserving procedures has not been as successful as was expected. Professionals thought that conservative surgery would reduce psychological morbidity, but there is little evidence to support this. Fifteen studies have shown that there is little difference in the psychological problems experienced by women who have radical surgery and those who have conservative surgery. Problems identified in both groups are fear of cancer, sexual dysfunction, altered body image and varying degrees of depression and anxiety. These effects were experienced in approximately 25–30% of patients.[14]

If patients request further help with coping with their disease, nurses can put them in contact with support groups. They could also use tools such as the Psychological Adjustment to Illness Scale (PAIS) and the Hospital Anxiety and Depressions Scale (HADS) to help detect depression or anxiety and make necessary referrals for clinical psychology or psychiatry support.[15]

NON-SURGICAL TREATMENT

Surgical treatment may be followed by an appropriate adjuvant therapy. This may take the form of chemotherapy, radiotherapy or hormone therapy.

Chemotherapy

In 1992 the Imperial Cancer Research Fund published an evaluation of adjuvant therapies based on results of studies from around the world. It concluded that adjuvant systemic therapy improves survival rates.[16]

Combination chemotherapy, such as cyclophosphomide, methotrexate and 5 fluorouracil (CMF) or IV adrayamyan and cyclophosomide, may be chosen for its association with reduced risk of early recurrence. Criteria such as tumour size, presence of positive nodes and histology are factors in the choice of chemotherapy used.

The effects of chemotherapy are well documented and the patient must be assessed for potential and actual effects of treatments. Physical side-effects include neutropenia, insomnia, sore mouth, constipation, diarrhoea, possible hair loss, nausea and vomiting. Nausea and vomiting can be controlled in most cases with the use of new antiemetics such as the 5HT3 receptor antagonists, for example, ondansatron. Symptom control is essential in helping patients cope with adjuvant therapy.[17]

Many patients find that alopecia can further damage their body image during chemotherapy. In a study reporting side-effects in patients undergoing 30 different chemotherapy regimes, 84% thought that alopecia was the most distressing symptom.[17]

Patients need to be aware of the likelihood of alopecia so they are less surprised and frightened when it occurs. Reassurance that their hair will grow back again is important, as is encouragement to get a good, well-fitting wig made prior to chemotherapy.

The psychological and social effects of chemotherapy may not be easy to recognise. These include reduced sex drive, altered perceptions of body image and withdrawal. A study of psychiatric morbidity in women who underwent a mastectomy and chemotherapy or mastectomy alone showed that significantly more women who received chemotherapy were rated as anxious or depressed.[17]

The long-term support of women undergoing treatments that have profound physical and psychological symptoms requires considerable knowledge and experience. It is in this area that the support or direct intervention of a specialist such as a breast care nurse may be required.

Radiotherapy

The majority of patients who have a wide local excision and some patients who have a mastectomy will have a course of radiotherapy. This usually means daily treatment over three to six weeks. Reactions to radiotherapy vary; some may fear that continuing treatment means that the cancer has not gone, while others will be reassured that it is a kind of insurance policy.

Side-effects include skin scaling, soreness, breast swelling, short-term fatigue, enlarged pores, erythema and dermatitis in the breast. Treatment may involve travelling a distance to specialist radiotherapy centres. This will involve extra expense. Financial help can be obtained by a grant from Cancer Relief Macmillan.

Hormone therapy

The specialised cells of the sex hormones and breasts are particularly dependent on the circulating sex hormones. It is now possible to test breast cancers for hormone sensitivity and to tailor adjuvant treatments to maximise the benefits for individual patients.

Women whose tumours contain oestrogen and progesterone receptors are likely to benefit from endocrine therapies while those with receptor-negative cancers are more likely to respond to chemotherapy, particularly if they are under 60.

A major factor in the increasing survival of breast cancer patients, particularly in the post-menopausal group, has been the development of increasingly sophisticated endocrine treatments. The first and still most widely used of these is the oestrogen antagonist tamoxifen citrate, which is the first-line drug of choice for adjuvant therapy in a majority of breast cancers.[16]

For the treatment of recurrent and advanced disease a number of new agents have been developed, particularly progestogens, aromatase inhibitors and a new generation of pure anti-oestrogens.[9] This is a rapidly expanding area of breast cancer treatment and shows much promise for further increased survival in the future.

THINKING POINTS

● What factors should be borne in mind when preparing the right environment for breaking bad news?
● What role can a nurse play in helping a woman with breast cancer make the best decision about the kind of surgery for her?

PART THREE

Revision notes

The UK has the highest breast cancer mortality rate in the world. It is the most commonly occurring carcinoma among British women, with 31 000 new diagnoses made in 1989.[1] Treatment, diagnosis and screening methods for breast cancer are undergoing constant development.

The exploration of the genetic causes of cancer generally, and breast cancer in particular, has the potential to improve screening and treatment.[18] Surgical interventions are being closely examined to ensure maximum effectiveness while reconstructive surgery is being advanced.

PATHOLOGY OF BREAST CANCER

Breast cancer is a systemic, rather than localised, disease in which micrometastases are frequently disseminated before the disease is detected. Screening is vitally important, but over 90% of breast cancers are initially detected by women themselves through breast self-examination.

In its early stages breast cancer is non-invasive, affecting mainly the ducts. Once a lesion has reached a size of 5mm there is a risk that it will invade the lymph nodes and thus enter the systemic circulation. Metastasis occurs most commonly in the lungs, bone, mediastinal lymph

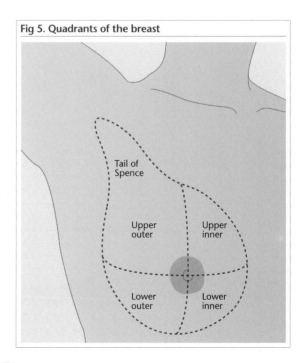

Fig 5. Quadrants of the breast

Tail of Spence

Upper outer

Upper inner

Lower outer

Lower inner

nodes or liver. Without treatment death may occur in three years. Tumours are most often situated in the upper outer quadrant of the breast. As it grows the tumour attaches to chest wall or overlying skin. Without treatment the surrounding tissues are invaded extending to the lymph glands of the axilla.

Clinical features
The first tangible sign is a mobile lump, which may either be painful or painless and may thicken. This can cause localised discomfort such as burning, stinging or aching. Shortening of the suspensory ligaments caused by fibrosis around the cancer may eventually cause dimpling or 'orange peel' appearance of the skin (Fig 2). The breast may appear asymmetric and elevated. Progress of the disease brings enlarged axillary nodes, tumour invasion of neighbouring tissue, ulceration and cachexia.

Tumour node metastasis (TNM) staging provides a means of describing and communicating the extent of disease progress and informs choice of appropriate treatment and likely prognosis (Table 2).

Prognosis
Breast cancer is unpredictable because it is influenced by factors such as hormone levels, immune response and host resistance. Where lymph nodes have not been involved prognosis is improved; however, the absence of nodes does not necessarily mean the absence of malignancy as growth may be microscopic. The extent of tumour spread at the time of treatment is more significant in prognosis.

RISK FACTORS

Breast cancer can be caused by a range of factors. The exact influence of some of these is yet to be firmly established. Some causative factors are environmental, such as exposure to radiation, some are related to lifestyle — being overweight, for example — while others are concerned with individual characteristics such as genetics.

Genetic predisposition
A family history involving dominant genes contributes to about 5% of breast cancers. In the UK that means about 1250 cases a year have a genetic cause.[18]

The most important genetic cause identified so far is the BRCa1 gene, which has been located on the long arm of chromosome 17 and accounts for 5% of all breast cancers. It occurs in about 45% of families where breast cancer is diagnosed under the age of 45 years. Possessing the gene carries an 80% risk of disease at the age of 80.

Other risk factors
The risk of developing breast cancer increases with age. Incidence is low below the age of 25, and increases towards menopause. There is a slight downward trend during the menopause, after which incidence rises again.[19]

Table 4. Factors to be included in patient assessment

● Beliefs and understanding of cancer and treatments

● Previous experience of cancer and treatments to elicit attitude and feelings

● The effects on body image, self-esteem and self-image

● The effects of diagnosis on relationships

● The effects on sexual functioning

● The effects on social and occupational activities

● Previous mental illness

● Religious and ethnic background

● Other variables that may contribute to the development of psychosocial problems

---

Other risk factors include:
● Previous history of breast cancer;
● Early onset of menarche, particularly when a regular menstrual cycle is established at an early age;
● Late onset of menopause (after the age of 55);
● Exposure to radiation, especially at a young age when breast tissue is developing;
● Previous history of benign breast disease;
● Having no children or having children after age 35;
● High bodyweight;
● Oral contraceptives use: subgroups of oral contraceptive users may have an increased risk; for example, women who have used oral contraception for several years before the age of 25 years and/or before the first full-term pregnancy;
● Hormone replacement therapy: studies into HRT as a risk factor have produced conflicting results. It may be some time before conclusive data becomes available about the common forms of HRT used in the UK.

TREATMENT
Surgical treatment now tends to be more conservative, with effort being made to minimise the disfigurement caused by procedures such as radical mastectomy. However, reports from randomised clinical trials comparing relapse-free intervals and survival in women with early-stage breast cancer removed by mastectomy or wide local excision demonstrated no differences in survival between the two groups.[4]

As a result some patients are encouraged to take part in decision-making about choices in surgical treatment. Most appreciate the opportunity to be involved in the decision process. Nurses can play a valuable role in helping patients weigh up the choices.

The degree of disfigurement following surgery can be compensated for, to some extent, by reconstructive surgery. This can be done immediately after mastectomy or after a period of rehabilitation.

Alternatively, a flap of skin, fat or muscle can be transferred from a donor site to the operative area. This involves grafting an island of latissimus dorsi muscle from the back, which is transplanted in the chest wall to form a reconstructed breast. Creating a tram flap involves transplanting abdominal skin and fat from the rectus abdominus muscle. This procedure has the advantage of bulk to form the whole of the breast without the need of an implant. Blood supply is re-established by reanastomosis of vessels from the operative area with those in the flap. A new nipple may be created with grafted tissue.

Surgical complications
Aside from the usual postsurgical complications, mastectomy wounds may be prone to inflammatory and circulatory problems. A gathering of exudate known as a seroma can occur in the space under the flaps of a mastectomy and can occur in wide excision surgery. Infection, necrosis of the flap and lymphoedema can also occur.

NURSING CARE AFTER SURGERY

Postoperative care is aimed at promoting freedom from pain and postsurgical complications. In the longer term, it is oriented towards supporting patients through alteration in body image and fear of cancer recurrence.

Pain relief is achieved through both analgesia and attention to position. Elevation of the arm affected by surgery will promote vascular and lymphatic drainage, controlling swelling and pain.

Circulation may be impeded by dressings and drains. The wound must be observed closely for accumulation of fluid under the skin flap.

After axillary surgery early use of the arm promotes fluid return and prevents swelling. The fingers and the wrist can be exercised straight away, with gentle use of the whole arm being encouraged soon after. More active exercises should be taught after the removal of sutures.

One risk is infection, especially where there is a stagnant collection of blood products in the wound. Infection can delay healing and increase the risk of lymphoedema. It is important therefore to promote cleanliness and freedom from irritation around the wound. This may be caused by creams or deodorants, for example.

NON-SURGICAL TREATMENT

Surgical treatment will be followed by an appropriate adjuvant therapy to ensure that all the carcinoma has been removed. This may take the form of chemotherapy, radiotherapy or hormone therapy.

Chemotherapy
Combination chemotherapy such as cyclophosphomide, methotrexate and 5 fluorouracil (CMF) reduces the risk of early recurrence. Physical side-effects include neutropenia, insomnia, sore mouth, constipation, diarrhoea, possible hair loss, nausea and vomiting. Chemotherapy also has psychological and social effects. These include a reduced sex drive, altered perceptions of body image and social withdrawal. A study of psychiatric morbidity in women who underwent mastectomy and chemotherapy or mastectomy alone showed that significantly more women who received chemotherapy were rated as anxious or depressed.[20] The long-term support of women undergoing treatment who have profound physical and psychological symptoms requires considerable specialised knowledge. It is in this area that the support or direct intervention of a specialist such as a breast-care nurse may be necessary.

Radiotherapy
Following a wide local excision most patients will have a course of radiotherapy. This usually means daily treatment over three to six weeks. Side-effects of radiotherapy include skin scaling, soreness, breast swelling, short-term fatigue, enlarged pores, erythema and dermatitis.

Endocrine therapy
Many breast cancers contain hormone receptors that render them dependent on circulating sex hormones for stimulation into growth. Consequently, manipulation of the hormone balance may retard development of the cancer cells or even cause a tumour to seem to melt away completely. The most common drug for this purpose is tamoxifen citrate but there are several others that may be used.

INVOLVEMENT OF THE BREAST-CARE NURSE

If survival rates in breast cancer are to be improved it is important that the available support should also be increased. A specialist nursing service provides practical information and support for patients and families affected by breast cancer. Approximately one third of patients with breast cancer will need specialised support or counselling in the early stages of treatment.[21] Such nursing input provides expertise, continuity and a means of coordinating care from other agencies. The diagnosis of breast cancer, which many patients regard as life-threatening, together with feeling stigmatised and rejected, are issues that confront all patients irrespective of the extent of surgical treatment or their age.

The capacity for patients and their families to respond to a diagnosis of cancer varies considerably. Much can depend on their prior experience of cancer, their ability to adapt and change, and the support they have within the extended family and community.

Intervention by a breast-care nurse can be appropriate at any time in a patient's and family's experience of cancer, but there are critical points for intervention:
● At time of diagnosis;
● During treatments;
● Three months after treatments have finished;
● At recurrence of breast cancer.

Research has shown that putting the onus on the patient to contact the breast-care nurse, usually three months after the initial diagnosis and finished treatments, is an effective strategy for improving patient support as

Fig 6. Breast reconstruction procedures

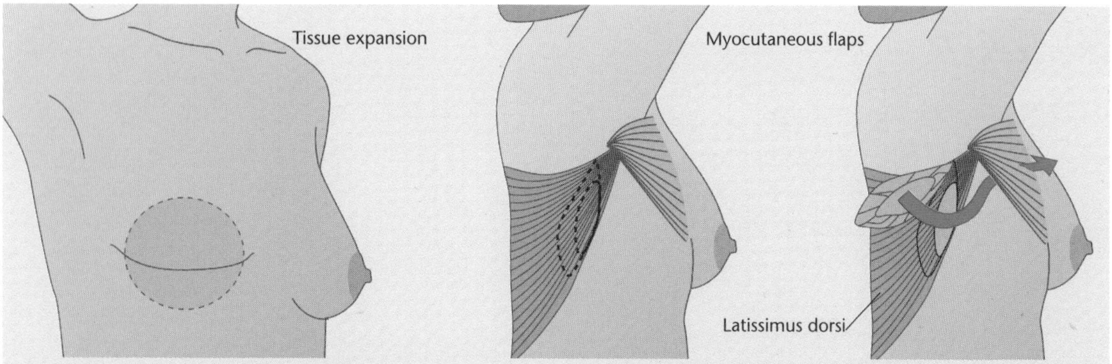

Tissue expansion

Myocutaneous flaps

Latissimus dorsi

A tissue expander is placed under the muscle, expanded with saline to create a pocket, then exchanged for an implant

A flap of skin, fat and muscle is transferred from the latissimus dorsi to the operative site, and blood supply is re-established with existing vessels

well as allowing the patient's independence. The nurse has a continuing role at times of crisis.

REFERENCES
1. Ursin, S., Bersteine, L. Pike, M.C. *Breast Cancer — Cancer Surveys 19/20: Trends in Cancer Incidence and Mortality.* London: Imperial Cancer Research Fund, 1994.
2. Kalache, A., Horton, D. *The Breast.* London: Longman, 1992.
3. Eeles, R. Developments in the study of familial breast cancer *Nursing Times* 1995; 91: 5, 29–33.
4. Henderson, B.E., Pike, M.G., Ross, R.K. *Epidemiology and Risk Factors in Breast Cancer: Diagnosis and Management.* Chichester: John Wiley, 1984.
5. Dixon, M., Sainsbury, R. *Diseases of the Breast.* Edinburgh: Churchill Livingstone, 1994.
6. Kvale, G., Heuche, I. A prospective study of reproductive factors and breast cancer. *American Journal of Epidemiology* 1987; 126: 842–845.
7. WHO. Collaborative study of neoplasia and steroid contraception. *Cancer* 1990; 61: 110–119.
8. UK National Case Control Study Group. Oral contraceptive use in breast cancer risk in young women. *Lancet* 1990; **335**: 1507–1509.
9. Collaborative Group on Hormone Factor in Breast Cancer. Breast Cancer and hormone replacement therapy: collaborative reanalysis of data from 51 epidemiological studies of 52,705 women without breast cancer. *Lancet* 1997; 350: 1047–1059.
10. Fallowfield, L.J., Baum, M., Maguire, G.P. Two effects of breast conservation on psychological morbidity. *British Medical Journal*, 1986; 293: 1311–1314.
11. Wilkinson, S., Maguire, G.P. A life after breast cancer. *Nursing Times*, 1988; 84: 40, 34–37.
12. Locker, A.P., Ellis, I.O., Morgan, D.A. Factors influencing local recurrence after excision and radiotherapy for primary breast cancer. *British Journal of Surgery* 1989; **76**: 890–894.
13. Cassilieth, B.R., Zupkiss, R.V., Sutton, S. et al. Preferences among cancer patients. *International Medicine* 1980; 92: 832–836.
14. Burt, K. The effects of cancer on body image and sexuality. *Nursing Times* 1995; 91: 7, 36–37.
15. Fallowfield, L.J. Assessment of quality of life in breast cancer. *Acta Oncology* 1995; 34: 689–694.
16. Early Breast Cancer Trialists Collaborative Group. Systemic treatment of early breast cancer by hormonal, cytotoxic or immune therapy. *Lancet* 1992; 339: 71–85
17. Colbourne, L. Patients' experiences of chemotherapy treatment. *Professional Nurse* 1995; 10; 7: 439–442.
18. Eeles, R. Developments in the study of familial breast cancer. *Nursing Times* 1995; 91: 5, 29–33.
19. Henderson, B.E., Pike, M.G., Ross, R.K. *Epidemiology and Risk Factors in Breast Cancer: Diagnosis and Management.* Chichester: John Wiley, 1984.
20. Wilkinson, S., Maguire, G.P. A life after breast cancer. *Nursing Times* 1988; 84: 40, 34–37.
21. Moorey, S. Adjuvant Psychological therapy for anxiety and depression. In: *A New Approach.* Oxford: Heinemann, 1993.

FURTHER READING
Denton, S. (ed) *Breast Cancer Nursing.* London: Chapman and Hall, 1996.
Dixon, M., Sainsbury, R. *Diseases of the Breast.* Edinburgh: Churchill Livingstone, 1994.
Fallowfield, L., Clark A. *Breast Cancer: The Experience of Illness.* London: Routledge, 1994.
Brennon, J. Altered body image. *Professional Nurse* 1994; 2: 299.

Useful addresses

BACUP, 3 Bath Place, Rivington Street, London, EC2A 3JR Tel: 0171-696 9003. Freephone helpline: 0800-181199
Breast Cancer Care, 210 New Kings Road, London SW6 4NZ Tel: 0171-384 2344. Freephone helpline: 0500-245345
Cancer Link, 17 Britannia Street, London WC1 9JN Tel: 0171-833 2451
Cancer Counselling Service Authority, London: 0171-696 9000 Glasgow: 0141-248 9277
Cancer Care , 21 Zetland Road, Redland, Bristol BS6 7AH Tel: 0117-942 7419
Cancer Relief Macmillan Fund, 15-19 Britten Street, London SW3 3T2 Tel: 0171-351 7811

BREAST CANCER

Breast cancer

Assessment

When you have read the unit and completed any further reading, you can use the questions below to test your understanding of the topic. Answers can be found on the next page

1 How many women in the UK die of breast cancer annually?

1 21 000
2 15 000
3 32 000
4 26 000

2 Which of the following countries has the highest mortality rate from breast cancer?

1 China
2 USA
3 UK
4 Sweden

3 What is the name of the main muscle anatomically associated with the breast?

1 Lateral dorsi
2 Pectoralis major
3 Pectoralis minor
4 The intercostal muscle

4 How many lobes are there in the breast?

1 4-6
2 15-20
3 30-40
4 40-50

5 The most common form of breast cancer is:

1 Ductal carcinoma *in situ*
2 Infiltrating lobular carcinoma
3 Infiltrating duct carcinoma
4 Tubular carcinoma

6 Adjuvant endocrine therapy is most often given using the drug

1 Megesterol acetate
2 Goserelin
3 Tamoxifen citrate
4 Formestane

7 The risk of breast cancer is increased if:

1 A woman has had more than one child
2 A woman has had no children
3 A woman has had a long break between
4 None of the above

8 The risk of breast cancer is increased if :

1 The onset of menarche is after the age of sixteen
2 There is an irregular menstrual cycle that lasts for more than five years
3 There is an irregular menstrual at an early age
4 There is early onset of menarche together with the early establishment of a regular menstrual cycle

9 Extensive surgery:

1 Is proven to be more successful in curing breast cancer than conservative surgery
2 Is less successful than conservative surgery in curing breast cancer
3 Has been found to be no more successful than conservative surgery in curing breast cancer
4 Is now popular because of the range of reconstructive surgery available

10 Chemotherapy can cause:

1 Painful reddening of the skin and nausea
2 Increased risk of infection, possible hair loss and dermatitis
3 Painful reddening of the skin, swelling in the breasts and nausea
4 Neutropenia, possible hair loss, nausea and vomiting

11 Radiotherapy can cause:

1 Photosensitivity, erythema and breast swelling
2 Erythema and breast swelling
3 Chronic fatigue, breast swelling and dermatitis
4 Soreness and scaling of the skin, fatigue during the treatment and dermatitis

12 **Mammography is the most effective investigation for breast cancer screening in:**

1	All age groups
2	Patients under the age of 50
3	Women after the menopause
4	None of the above

13 **Breast cancer:**

1	Spreads easily throughout the body
2	Is confined to one area only
3	Is only detectable by X-ray and ultrasound
4	Is rarely found in those over the age of 30

14 **Use of the oral contraceptive pill:**

| 1 | Is linked with increased breast cancer |
| 2 | May increase the risk of breast cancer in the presence of a strong family history |

| 3 | Is a risk only if used for more than 10 years |
| 4 | Is in no way linked to increased risk |

15 **After mastectomy the wound may be prone to infection; this risk can be reduced by:**

1	Advising the patient to keep the skin around the wound moisturised
2	Advising patients to wash the wound with soap for two weeks after surgery
3	Advising patients to avoid irritating the wound, by using underarm deodorants, for instance
4	Advising the patients to wear loose clothing for one month after surgery

---

ANSWERS

Breast cancer

1: How many women in the UK die of breast cancer annually:
2) 15 000

2: Which of the following countries has the highest mortality rate from breast cancer:
3) UK

3: What is the name of the main muscle anatomically associated with the breast:
2) Pectoralis major

4: How many lobes are there in the breast?
2) 15–20

5: The most common form of breast cancer is:
3) Infiltrating duct carcinoma

6: Adjuvant endocrine therapy is most often given using the drug:
3) Tamoxifen citrate

7: The risk of breast cancer is increased if?
2) A woman has had no children

8: The risk of breast cancer is increased if?
4) There is early onset of menarche together with the early establishment of a regular menstrual cycle

9: Extensive surgery:
3) Has been found to be no more successful than conservative surgery

10: Chemotherapy can cause:
4) Neutropenia, possible hair loss, nausea and vomiting

11: Radiotherapy can cause:
4) Soreness and scaling of the skin, fatigue during the treatment and dermatitis

12: Mammography is the most effective investigation for breast cancer screening:
3) Women after the menopause

13: Breast cancer:
1) Spreads easily through the body

14: Use of the oral contraceptive pill:
2) May increase the risk of breast cancer in the presence of strong family history

15: After mastectomy the wound may be prone to infection; this can be reduced by:
3) Advising patients to avoid irritating the wound, by using underarm deodorants, for instance

Digestive tract cancers

Knowledge for practice

In this look at common gastrointestinal cancers we will use Carper's patterns of knowing as the framework within which to organise and present the knowledge for practice and role of the nurse.[1] This is because no two patients, cancers or nurses are the same, and a prescriptive list of ways to do things means nurses and patients must make sense of the different sources of knowledge and apply it to their unique experience (Box 1).

Carper identifies four patterns of knowing, or approaches to knowledge, that nurses will need to help them to practice effectively.[1] No one pattern is more important than another, but combined they help the nurse organise his or her knowledge for practice (Box 2).

Malignancies of the gastrointestinal (GI) tract account for 26% of total malignancies diagnosed in England and Wales.[2] Nurses involved with caring for adult patients will encounter people with a cancer in the GI tract in various clinical areas. A background of factual knowledge for nursing patients with this disease will help practitioners to develop their nursing care appropriately.

This section provides empirical information about commonly occurring GI tract malignancies and the moral difficulties nurses may experience when nursing this group of patients.

The incidence of GI tract cancers around the world varies. Studies of migrant populations demonstrate assimilation of the migrant population's incidence rate with that of the indigenous group within one or two generations. This and the overall association of these malignancies with ageing indicate the undeniable link with environmental factors. The environment of the digestive tract is comprised of the food and drink ingested over a period of time, and it would appear that both quality and quantity are factors.

The most common GI tract malignancy in the UK and the developed world is colorectal cancer. It is the second most commonly diagnosed cancer in men and women. This and more commonly occurring malignant tumours in other parts of the GI tract will be considered, namely the oesophagus, stomach and pancreas.

PRESENTATION

The GI tract is unpredictable in its habits with occasional bouts of nausea, vomiting, diarrhoea, unusual flatulence or odd pains. Commonly this is due to an unknown pathogen or mild abuse of food or alcohol and does not present a lasting problem. Consequently, it is often some time before people experiencing altered bowel habit present to a doctor complaining of persistent symptoms. Symptoms are likely to be related to problematic swallowing, excessive belching and heartburn or retrosternal pain in cancers of the oesophagus or stomach.

Box 1. Aetiology of cancers in the gastrointestinal system

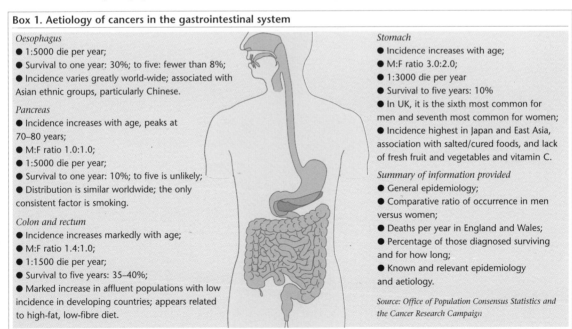

Oesophagus
- 1:5000 die per year;
- Survival to one year: 30%; to five: fewer than 8%;
- Incidence varies greatly world-wide; associated with Asian ethnic groups, particularly Chinese.

Pancreas
- Incidence increases with age, peaks at 70–80 years;
- M:F ratio 1.0:1.0;
- 1:5000 die per year;
- Survival to one year: 10%; to five is unlikely;
- Distribution is similar worldwide; the only consistent factor is smoking.

Colon and rectum
- Incidence increases markedly with age;
- M:F ratio 1.4:1.0;
- 1:1500 die per year;
- Survival to five years: 35–40%;
- Marked increase in affluent populations with low incidence in developing countries; appears related to high-fat, low-fibre diet.

Stomach
- Incidence increases with age;
- M:F ratio 3.0:2.0;
- 1:3000 die per year
- Survival to five years: 10%
- In UK, it is the sixth most common for men and seventh most common for women;
- Incidence highest in Japan and East Asia, association with salted/cured foods, and lack of fresh fruit and vegetables and vitamin C.

Summary of information provided
- General epidemiology;
- Comparative ratio of occurrence in men versus women;
- Deaths per year in England and Wales;
- Percentage of those diagnosed surviving and for how long;
- Known and relevant epidemiology and aetiology.

Source: Office of Population Consensus Statistics and the Cancer Research Campaign

---

Presentation may be more acute with, for example, haematemesis. Other symptoms are likely to have been present for some time.

In cancer of the pancreas patients commonly present with more generalised symptoms of lethargy and with obstructive jaundice together with itching and dry skin. Back pain is also a common feature, particularly in carcinoma of the body of the pancreas. All patients with upper GI tract malignancy will describe significant weight loss over a few months or even weeks where there is an obstructive lesion.

The signs of malignancy are similar to those of indigestion but also include increasing persistence of altered symptoms over time with weight loss. Any new bleeding should be immediately investigated regardless of whether it has been experienced in the past.

Cancers of the colon and rectum are initially symptomless. Weight loss is a classic sign but occurs some months or years after tumour initiation. Altered bowel habit is not uncommon but may take any form: distension; alternating constipation and loose stools; diarrhoea; or more frequent defecation. Increased flatulence and tenesmus (wanting to defecate with nothing there), increased production of mucous, and/or blood may be described.

Bleeding from the rectum may be visible or occult. If visible, it may be associated with piles. Occult bleeding is unknown to the patient. Weight loss and anaemia may provide the first clue to the problem, particularly in older people. Some may present acutely with bowel obstruction or perforation which may be confused with diverticular disease.

AETIOLOGY

In seeking the cause of a disease, prevention or cure are the real goals. Patients and their relatives often enquire as to what could have caused them to become ill, partly to try to protect themselves in the future, and partly to supply an explanation for the situation they are now in. There is no definite answer — however, there are clues about possible causes.

External factors
In oesophageal cancer, different worldwide incidence indicates dietary environmental carcinogens. In the developed world there is a link with alcohol and tobacco use. Other risks include chronic acid reflux causing inflammatory cellular changes (Barrett's oesophagus) or achalasia, or malnutrition.[3]

Recently it has been confirmed that chronic growth of the bacteria *Helicobacter pylori* in the stomach predisposes patients to ulceration and carcinoma.[4]

Indicators for pancreatic cancer are difficult to ascertain as patients are ill when first referred and too few survive to gain substantive information. Smoking and dietary factors have been implicated.

Indicative habits in colorectal cancer are also related to diet, particularly the combination of a high-fat diet, too many processed or refined foods and lack of exercise. Leading a more active lifestyle and consuming fresh fruit and vegetables — particularly curciferous vegetables such as cabbage, broccoli and spinach, may confer protection. Ulcerative colitis patients are likely to develop carcinoma at one or more sites in the colorectum as time from diagnosis increases, particularly is there has been severe ulceration and a large area has been affected.

In coming to terms with a new diagnosis people inevitably wonder 'why me ?' and will be seeking answers to the question. General advice about healthy eating and lifestyle changes is likely to be more helpful than a list of items which may have led to their cancer.

Genetics
Recent advances in medical genetics have established links between inherited genetic characteristics and development of cancers during life. Within gastroenterology there is known inherited susceptibility in colorectal cancer with possible links in some cases to stomach cancer.

Colorectal cancer is best understood alongside several inherited conditions leading to development of malignancy.

High-risk groups for colorectal cancer include those with familial adenomatous polyposis syndromes — familial polyposis coli, Turcot's or Gardner's syndromes. Among other signs these individuals inherit the tendency to develop colonic polyps, one or more of which will almost certainly become malignant by 35 years. The other inherited conditions are the Lynch or 'cancer family' or hereditary non polyposis colorectal cancers syndromes. In Lynch I syndrome there is an inherited tendency to develop colorectal cancer, whereas Lynch II results in a susceptibility to adenocarcinoma of the breast, colon, rectum, uterus or other sites.

The majority of colorectal cancers occur spontaneously though there is increasing evidence which indicates that DNA coding is a contributing factor. It is known that people with a parent or sibling with colorectal cancer have an increased risk of developing the disease. The younger the patient at diagnosis, the more likely a genetic component, particularly where no other risk factors are known to be involved.

Fig 1. Distribution of cancers within the colon

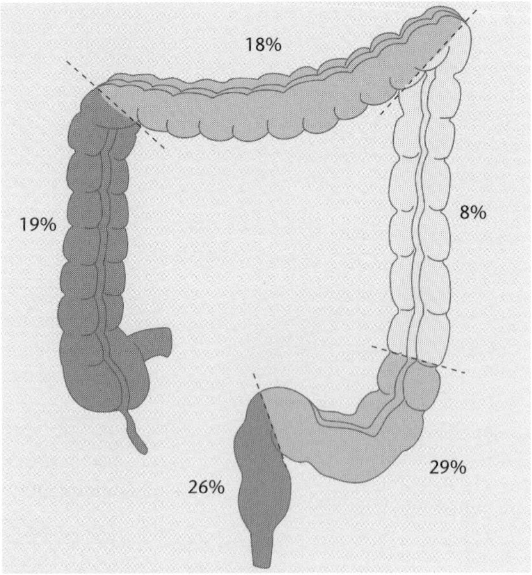

Implications of hereditary illness

People are increasingly aware of the potential for inheriting a tendency to develop cancer. The psychological implications on diagnosis are thus more significant. Nurses need to be aware of the implications when the possibility of an inherited syndrome is involved in diagnosis.

If a genetic component to the patient's disease has been confirmed, the patient may fear that children and grandchildren or siblings will succumb to the same fate he or she is currently faced with, both physically and emotionally. Fear and anger may be exacerbated by his or her powerlessness to change or avoid the situation. Guilt about the legacy to be handed on will be a factor, although it may be obscured by other emotions or coping strategies. Some people exhibit a surprising optimism. They may even appear unable to accept or discuss the diagnosis and its implications at all, leaving an increased burden on other family members.

With more than one member of the family involved, stress can be placed on everyone, and it is often nursing staff, in close proximity to those involved, who may witness or take the brunt of turbulent emotions. Nurses need to be able to have some understanding of what is involved in order that they may calmly support and inform all parties concerned with a recent diagnosis of genetically determined cancer syndromes.

It is invaluable for nurses to have considered their own concerns and anxieties about such a situation were it to happen to them. Personal beliefs and feelings will be integral to any nurse's approach to patients, whether wittingly or not, thus, practitioners must be aware of their own feelings in order to deal objectively and sensitively with clients. The inherited syndromes by virtue of their predictability are suitable for screening to prevent development of malignancy in the future.

In the UK colorectal cancer is usually the only GI tract malignancy considered for regular screening. In addition people who have other predisposing conditions for colorectal cancer will usually be screened for early stages of disease.

INVESTIGATIONS AND STAGING

On diagnosis with carcinoma, further information is required to establish the stage of the disease. Staging is a framework to describe the type, invasion or size, lymph node involvement and distant spread of a tumour. This information indicates prognosis, appropriate treatment or symptom control.

Patients set enormous store by the numerous, often degrading, tests they are subjected to — inevitably hoping for better news, and all those involved wait anxiously for results. In general, most investigations will include insertion of instrumentation into the oral or anal orifices. This is an extremely unpleasant invasion for the patient, whether or not sedation is used.

While it is not appropriate to give definitive results before final reports are made, experienced nurses may feel it suitable to broach the subject of possible findings with individual patients in certain circumstances either to allay fears or to allow maximum time for bad news to be confronted. This should always be in consultation and agreement with the medical staff responsible for diagnosis and suggested treatment options.

Investigative procedures

Generally all tumours of the digestive tract will be diagnosed with endoscopy and/or contrast radiography, usually barium swallow or enema. Upper GI tract malignancies may be confirmed with endoscopy, at which point brushings of mucosal cells and tissue biopsies are taken and sent for histology reporting.

In pancreatic cancer, endoscopic retrograde cholangiopancreatography (ERCP) will demonstrate any ductal obstruction with contrast dye, and facilitate both biopsy and relief of jaundice with stenting of the ampulla. Most colorectal cancers are initially diagnosed with rigid or flexible sigmoidoscopy; 50% of cancers occur in the rectum and sigmoid colon within reach of a sigmoidoscope (50cms in length).[5]

Alternatively, colonoscopy (150cm length) may be indicated for higher tumours, and in this situation, a double contrast barium enema is a useful tool. Radiologically, ultrasound, computed tomography scanning and magnetic resonance imaging may be used to provide further information about extent of tumour bulk or metastasis (spread to lymph nodes or other organs).

Recently the use of intralumenal ultrasound (a scanning probe passed into oesophagus or rectum as an endoscope) has been developed to provide information about the extent of invasion into the gut wall of oesophageal and colorectal tumours. Final evaluation may only be possible with surgery, although for some patients this may not be appropriate.

TREATMENT AND PROGNOSIS

Nurses play a vital role in the decision about treatment options, according to their knowledge of the patient and the patient's need for advocacy. Patients require increased support and advice in such situations as decision making can be confused by an anxious state of mind.

Difficult circumstances often surround decision making, which may then have an effect on treatment plans from a moral stance as well as a physical one, given that survival from digestive tract cancer is low. While all involved want the best result for the patient, this may not necessarily be measured in length of time, and should always be considered in terms of quality of life.

Surgical intervention

In all the carcinomas described, surgical intervention is the primary consideration, particularly if staging indicates a potential for cure. In almost all cases this is a daunting prospect as surgery is likely to be extensive. The patient may be unwell beforehand, and potentially highly dependent and at risk from postoperative complications for some weeks following the operation.

In most surgical interventions aimed at curative resection there is likely to be significant anatomical reconstruction with impacts on the patient's body image and future lifestyle. From limiting the capacity of the stomach and permanently altering eating habits, through to forming a temporary or permanent colostomy, the implications of surgery can be immense.

Combined treatment approaches

Approaches to active treatment often combine surgery with radiotherapy or chemotherapy or both. Pre- and post-operative radiotherapy, to shrink tumours before surgery or minimise metastatic spread, may be used. Alternatively, radiotherapy may be useful in palliation, particularly in oesophageal or rectal cancers. It is not felt to be particularly helpful in pancreatic cancer and special care is required in gastric cancers to avoid excessive damage to the stomach or surrounding organs.

Chemotherapy is advancing and recent trials have shown combinations of cytotoxic drug regimes in conjunction with surgery to offer better survival rates, particularly for colorectal cancers. The options for treatment are increasingly varied. Toxicity of radiotherapy and chemotherapy vary according to the intensity of treatment used or the combination of drugs used.

Improving the quality of life with continuing care and symptom control is often the preferential option. Metastatic disease is usually to the liver via lymph glands in the surrounding mesentery though it may be to the lungs or brain in upper digestive tract cancers; hepatic carcinoma is rarely due to a primary growth.

Relief of distressing symptoms such as nausea, vomiting, the effects of jaundice, bowel obstruction and pain are now paramount concerns and are all controllable with advice from palliative-care specialists.

Caring for patients dying of GI tract carcinoma may be both distressing and rewarding for all involved. Being in a position to help a patient and his or her family through such an experience both physically and emotionally requires continuity and caring. For nurses who have known the patient for a long period of time, it is often painful but appropriate to continue the supportive and caring relationship to its end.

THINKING POINTS

● Towards what kind of resources and information would you point a patient to help him or her improve their diet?
● What kinds of information and support are needed by someone who is told that they have a genetic predisposition to cancer?

PART TWO

Role of the nurse

No two patients, gastrointestinal cancers or indeed nurses are exactly the same. A prescriptive list of ways to do things or typical descriptions of the disease progression require nurses and patients to make sense of and link different sources of knowledge to their own experience (Box3).

This section explores the art of nursing and the use of self, or personal knowledge, when caring for patients with gastrointestinal (GI) cancer. Fundamental to this approach is placing the patient centrally and looking at the experience from his or her perspective, and seeing what issues are raised for nurses involved in the care of these patients. This will inevitably lead into identifying the role of the nurse.

Box 3. Nursing contribution over the course of the disease

Time continuum of disease process →

Day one	Weeks/months				Up to a year	Years	Three to five years+		
First symptoms	GP	Hospital OPD	Investigations	Diagnosis and treatment / Surgery	Recovery period	Monitoring	Reoccurence	Continuing care	Death

Nurses potentially involved in care

	Practice nurse	Clinic nurse	X-ray endoscopic nurse	Pre-admission clinic nurse	Primary/ named nurse	District/ stoma nurse	Endoscopy clinic nurse	District nurse Macmillan nurse

The structure used to describe this is the time continuum from the patient's point of view of the disease process. Plotted against this continuum are the key moments for the patient, from diagnosis to cure or death, and different nurses who come into contact with the patient and his or her family at different stages.

The diagnosis may last for the rest of the patient's life. GI cancer mostly affects men and women in their 50s and 60s facing normal social changes and upheaval such as children growing up and leaving home, and retirement. The impact of diagnosis, treatment and continuing review of the disease then becomes a significant feature over the years to come. What must be remembered is the impact of this on close family members — especially spouses and children.

The second feature from the review of the time continuum is the number of different nurses a patient may encounter in the course of diagnosis, treatment and care. With patients meeting so many different nurses it becomes clear how potentially confusing it can be — not least working out what each nurse does that is different from the others but also the lack of continuity in nursing care and the potential for conflicting information, advice and support. In the light of these two points, the review of the nurse's role picks up on four key activities nurses can and should see as their role. These are: effective use of self in one-to-one interaction with patients; skills of assessment; interpersonal skills of information giving, listening and counselling; and team-working skills.

USE OF SELF

The commitment by individual nurses to their relationships with patients is integral to nursing. However, nurses should take time to develop a clear awareness of themselves and their skills, and be honest both with themselves and their patients as to how this commitment works out in practice. For example, a ward or district nurse who has recently been bereaved is probably not able to work with individual families exploring this subject.[6]

The nurse also needs to recognise the nature of his or her relationships. For example, nurses working in endoscopy clinics will have only a brief time to establish relationships with individual patients, although they may encounter patients briefly months or years later as they return to the clinic for review. In contrast, ward and district nurses' relationships may last for weeks and months and those in clinical speciality roles, such as stoma nurses and Macmillan nurses, may find relationships lasting over months and years. It is important, therefore, that nurses are realistic about what therapeutic work can be achieved in the available time. Helping someone tackle his or her marital relationships during a short period of time is not realistic and can in some circumstances cause more problems than were started with.

ASSESSMENT

A patient may be assessed a number of times by different nurses. The nurse needs good assessment skills and a clear picture of the key issues that need to be reviewed. Appropriate choice of a nursing model and its careful application is important. No particular model is recommended, rather, the nurses involved should make that decision. What needs to be considered is the ease with which such assessments are transferable and can be updated as further encounters with the patient occur. This allows nurses to identify the use of coping mechanisms and adaptation to the impact of diagnosis and treatment over time.

Assessment should include the social and biographical details, review of physical signs and symptoms, the views, concerns and feelings the patient has regarding the diagnosis and what support, both personal and external, the patient has in managing this new life crisis.

For example, consider the assessment by the clinic or endoscopy nurse who may be involved with the doctor in the initial confirmation of the cancer diagnosis. Nurses are involved in investigations such as upper gastrointestinal endoscopy, sigmoidoscopy, colonoscopy, either in outpatient clinics or endoscopy units (Fig 2). Often after an investigation is carried out the doctor confirms the diagnosis and the nurse stays with the patient as he or she starts absorbing the news.

The following discussion might then tackle issues such as whether he or she thought it might be cancer, how he or she recognised the symptoms and the period of time over which he or she debated about seeking medical advice, whether he or she has people with them today in the clinic to go home with, what he or she will say to the children? These and many other questions are raised. The clinic nurse has an important role in using this time effectively with patients.

Opportunities for assessment

Nurses need to be skilled at rapidly developing trusting relationships with patients. Initial barriers may be broken down by the intimate investigations many gastrointestinal cancers involve. For example, enemas are required prior to sigmoidoscopy. The nurse will have been in support of the patient throughout the procedure. It is therefore appropriate that subsequent conversations with the nurse will explore the impact of diagnosis and immediate concerns. So much valuable information is available to nurses at this time but often it is lost.

More formal, documented assessments are carried out when the treatment phase begins on an in-patient basis. This is most common for surgery but may also include radiotherapy. Assessment at this stage should occur promptly although some patients may wait weeks or occasionally months (depending on waiting lists) from the initial hospital clinic appointment.

Significant adjustment will have taken place in that time. If the diagnosis has not been confirmed the patient may display significant anxiety and be reluctant to discuss the diagnosis in the hope it will not be confirmed. However, it would be helpful for nurses to know the precise language and phrases used by health-care professionals earlier in the patient's care. Ward nurses have little time with patients prior to surgery and, for this reason, can find it difficult to establish trusting relationships with them before theatre in order to explore this comfortably. Increasingly, the pre-admission arrangements, which largely involve pre-clerking and the practical considera-

tions of safe preparation, mean this aspect of care can become very fragmented if documentation is not maintained by the relevant nurses involved.

The assessment at this stage requires clear documentation of who said what, when and what the nurse's assessment of the patient's views and concerns are, so the primary or named nurse in the ward can build on this as his or her relationship with the patient develops.

Following the major treatment phase patients may require further nursing support at home. District nurses and some clinical nurse specialists will be involved, and a holistic assessment of the patient and his or her family will need to be undertaken. Some nurses are able to take advantage of patient-held nursing notes as these are with the patients at home.

However, for those who cannot, they are starting from scratch again, building up the relationship, assessing the physical impact surgery has had and what stage in the recovery has been achieved. Returning home to family and friends, patients still have significant physical recovery to complete, such as returning to normal eating and drinking patterns, regular bowel activities and, for those with new stomas, getting into a different routine.

Patients may be concerned about confidently recognising new sensations and functions and accepting them as normal, and worrying about new symptoms being attributable to cancer.

From the psychological perspective, the nurse needs to assess how the patient is getting on with living with the diagnosis, settling down any changed or disturbed family relationships and seeking to avoid further problems with cancers by looking at changes in lifestyle; for example, giving up smoking, accommodating the recommended dietary advice and learning how to cope better with stress.

INTERPERSONAL SKILLS

Three main interpersonal skills are of particular importance for the GI cancer care nurse, namely information-giving, listening and counselling.

Information-giving

It is vital that good-quality information is available to patients and their families when required. Responsibility rests with doctors and nurses to ensure that factual information is presented clearly in straightforward, easily understood language. A number of information centres provide general background information which patients, their families and friends may find helpful; for example the British Association for Cancer United Patients (BACUP). None the less, the information that patients receive which is specific to them and which they receive from their nurse and doctor will usually add to their confidence. The nurse should take steps to achieve the following: be sure the language and terms used are understood and familiar to the patients and his or her family; avoid hiding behind medical and nursing jargon; be con-

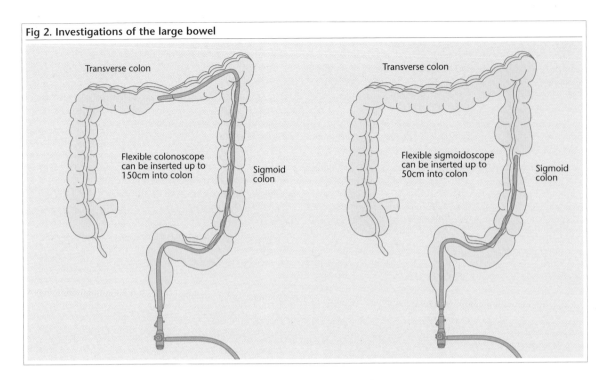

Fig 2. Investigations of the large bowel

Transverse colon

Flexible colonoscope can be inserted up to 150cm into colon

Sigmoid colon

Transverse colon

Flexible sigmoidoscope can be inserted up to 50cm into colon

Sigmoid colon

sistent in use of the words and phrases used; be with the doctor when information is given so as to be sure of what was said and reinforce or explain further with confidence.

The artistry the nurse displays in tailoring the information given in terms of language — the words and phrases, the timing of when to discuss aspects such as prognosis or recurrence of symptoms and the implications, when to include family members and when to continue with one-to-one conversations — is a key feature to this nursing work. For example, some patients with young family members have considerable concern about what to tell their children and how much to tell them. Often patients value talking through the options and rehearsing this.

None the less the personal impact this can have makes it difficult to talk frankly in front of spouses. Here the nurse can ensure one-to-one opportunities are made available for patients as well as family discussions. Similarly, patients will want to hear about how other people cope in order to see whether their experience is different or the same. The nurse, therefore, needs to be able to give this kind of information as well as the more factual information regarding incidence and aetiology.

Listening
Inevitably the quality of listening the nurse is able to achieve and maintain is significant in helping him or her to be an effective communicator. Some of the changes and achievements a patient makes in coming to terms and living with his or her diagnosis are very subtle and without active listening these changes can be overlooked. There is

also the danger that nurses continue talking with a patient and sometimes do not use silence as a means of communicating. Sometimes just the nurse being there is important for the patient; you do not have to come up with an answer or solution.

Counselling
Listening leads into the area of counselling, which many see as integral to the nurses role. Basic counselling skills are taught in pre-registration courses but sometimes more sophisticated skills are required and the nurse may need to think about taking further training for this kind of work. None the less, an awareness of recognising patients who are in difficulty and referring to more appropriate counsellors may well be indicated. It is not appropriate to enter into a counselling relationship with a patient with whom you are going to spend a short time.

This will limit the work you can carry out with them as their primary/named nurse and there may be difficulties in determining priorities of care. In some respects the district nurses and clinical nurse specialists, for example, stoma care nurse or Macmillan nurses may be better placed, if not more skilled in taking this work forward. So caution is required in taking on a formal counselling role but in some situations it may be appropriate.

Survival rates
Survival in GI tract cancers is poor, particularly in cancer of the oesophagus, stomach and pancreas. Recently diagnosed patients may exhibit a fighting spirit while simulta-

neously struggling with fear.

To be diagnosed with cancer can be a shock. It can cause guilt — particularly if the person has dependents or if he or she had ignored advice to see a doctor. The ideal of self-preservation is shattered for all those involved, and guilt and anger may be stirred up, with potentially serious consequences for family relationships. Anger may be compounded by medical professionals underestimating the anxiety caused.

Team-working skills
As the time continuum demonstrates there are a number of different nurses involved and at each stage there may well be different doctors.

Nurses must tackle the lack of continuity for patients. Improved documentation in the form of patient-held notes will help but there also needs to be a clearer awareness and good working relationships from the groups alongside each other on the continuum. In particular, the clinic, endoscopy and pre-admission nurses need to be sure of new working practices and use each other in ensuring patient-centred care is achieved.

Similarly ward nurses and district nurses who have both encountered changes in their working practices over recent years need to work hard providing seamless care between hospital and home by being quite clear of each other's changing working practices.

The most consistent person as far as the patient is concerned is the consultant and the GP, but junior doctors move around and over a period of years they will change. The nurse therefore needs to able to make contact and establish good rapport with senior doctors, being aware of the depth of knowledge a consultant may have about his or her patient.

Being able to present your concerns confidently and to identify possible actions coupled with a clear understanding of the roles others have within your team is vital. Negotiating referral to other members of the team as and when necessary is important.

As has been outlined, the nurse's role is key to the patient's experience of living with a cancer of the digestive system.

The number of different nurses involved over the typical timescale of the disease are many and varied. Nurses need to work hard at maintaining effective communication between themselves and with others involved if they are to avoid omitting or duplicating care.

THINKING POINTS

● How effective is information-giving for patients in your clinical area? How could it be improved?
● Incomplete bowel preparation can result in delayed diagnosis. What factors result in ineffective bowel preparation? How can these be remedied?

PART THREE

Revision notes

Gastrointestinal (GI) tract cancer incidence varies around the world, in different populations and ethnic groups. The major influence appears to be environmental. In the case of the GI tract, the environment is what one puts into it — that is food and drink, and the chemical reactions of these substances with the tissues lining the gut. Hence, in countries with higher incidences of specific GI tract cancers, there seem to be associations with dietary patterns and lifestyles.

Colorectal cancer (Fig 3) is the most common of the gastrointestinal cancers in the UK, and the UK has one of the highest incidences in the world. The overall survival figures for colorectal cancers are 35–40% at five years. (It should be noted that these are the best survival figures for all the cancers of the digestive tract). The prognosis is worse for patients with malignancy of the oesophagus, stomach and pancreas.[7] Given the overall prevalence of these cancers in our society, this is a considerable problem and one that has not improved noticeably within the past 30 years. Part of the reason for poor survival is that the symptoms of any of the GI tract cancers can be confused by patients as attributable to more common and simple complaints. It is often only the persistent nature of the problem that prompts a patient to seek an initial consultation with his or her GP. However, by the time symptoms have persisted, even only for a few months, it is likely that the cancer will be somewhat advanced and the potential for cure significantly reduced.

PRESENTATION

Upper GI tract symptoms may include some or all of the following: difficulties with swallowing (gradually worsening in time from solids to liquids); excessive belching; persistent heartburn and/or retrosternal pain; haemetemesis; itching or dry skin (jaundice in bile duct obstruction is associated with carcinoma of the head of pancreas); and weight-loss increasing exponentially over time.

Lower GI tract cancer symptoms may include some or all of the following:
● Altered bowel habit;
● Distension;
● Alternating constipation with loose stools;
● Diarrhoea;
● Not needing to defecate for long periods of time;
● Increased flatulence;
● Tenesmus (wanting to defecate without any faeces in the rectum);
● Passing mucous rectally;
● Bleeding from the rectum — there may be visible or occult in the stools;
● Weight loss over months;
● Anaemia.

The public is generally much less aware of digestive tract cancers than other diseases and it is not difficult to understand why — people may not be accustomed to discussing their guts and their behaviour in a serious manner, and will avoid confronting a long-standing problem because of embarrassment and the fear of wasting doctors' time. Patients and relatives should be reassured about seeking early referral if they are encountering problems as listed above, or if they fall into one of the groups at particular risk and eligible for screening.

The nurse's dilemma is how to approach such patients, knowing that the prognosis is likely to be poor but being in a position to discuss openly the prospects for the remainder of the patient's life with them or their family. However, whether or not the need to initiate discussion about the future is apparent, a sensitive and holistic approach to nursing is always appropriate.

In areas of practice where these patients are more commonly encountered, such as gastroenterology clinics or surgical wards, much may be gained from professional discussion groups. These may be formal support groups for staff or multidisciplinary conferences to discuss specific cases and plan the team's approach to their care.

GENETICS

In the UK colorectal cancer has been identified as having predisposing conditions. These include:
● People with a parent or sibling with colorectal cancer;
● Known occurrence of inherited familial adenomatous polyposis syndrome;
● Inherited Lynch syndromes (adenocarcinoma syndromes);
● Ulcerative colitis.

All patients within these categories should be offered regular screening to ensure early diagnosis and thus prompt treatment or even prevention of colorectal cancer. Some colorectal cancers are thought to have a pre-malignant stage — the benign adenomatous polyp. Left in the bowel these can develop and become malignant and invasive.

If found at the benign stage they can be removed without recurrence or malignancy. This may be done at the time of diagnosis with colonoscopy without requiring major surgery.

SCREENING

Screening a population for a disease is aimed at reducing deaths from the disease, and carries certain conditions. The principles of screening are:
● The condition screened for must be an important health problem;
● There should be an acceptable treatment for patients with recognised disease;
● Facilities for diagnosis and treatment should be available in sufficient quantity to meet the demands required as a result of screening case-finding;
● The disease should have a recognisable latent or early symptomatic stage;
● The natural course of the disease, including the latent phase to declared disease, should be adequately understood;
● There should be a suitable test or examination;
● This test must be acceptable to the population;
● There should be an agreed policy on whom to treat as patients;
● The cost of case-finding (including diagnosis and treatment of patients) should be economically balanced in relation to possible expenditure on medical care as a whole;
● Case-finding should be a continuing process and not a once-for-all process.[8]

Endoscopy
Curable stages are known in colorectal and stomach cancer but because they occur within the abdomen and pelvis they are impossible to detect at an early enough stage without endoscopy.

It is not feasible to endoscope the whole population over 50 years of age, the optimum length of time between endoscopies has not been established, but what is certainly beyond doubt is that this is unlikely to be acceptable to most people, and is excessively expensive in terms of staff, equipment and resources for treating the increased numbers of patients that would be found by screening.

In Japan screening for stomach cancer is done in some areas as it is such a large problem; similarly, some groups are screened for oesophageal cancer in China.

In the UK trials for the effectiveness of screening for colorectal cancer have been going on for some years. It is felt that death rates from the disease are likely to be reduced by screening the population aged over 50 but the most effective and cost-effective method of doing this has yet to be agreed; that is, occult blood testing or sigmoidoscopy.

INVESTIGATIONS AND TREATMENT

Investigating symptoms is intended to establish a diagnosis. However, staging is also important to establish progression of the disease and to determine the most effective treatment for the patient. Nearly all investigations involve instrumentation of oral or anal orifices and include the following:
● Oesophagoscopy or gastroscopy — with brushings of mucosal cells and tissue biopsy for histology;
● Endoscopic retrograde cholangio-pancreatography (ERCP);
● Contrast radiography — barium swallow; barium enema; or double-contrast barium enema;
● Sigmoidoscopy — rigid or flexible to a height of 50cm within the sigmoid colon (50% of colorectal cancers occur within the sigmoid colon or rectum); tissue samples can be biopsied and polyps can be removed;
● Colonoscopy — complete examination of the interior of the colon and rectum; biopsies and polypectomy are possible at this stage;
● Ultrasound (abdominal or endoscopic);
● Computer-aided tomography (CAT) or magnetic resonance imaging (MRI) scanning — particularly for assessing spread before and after treatment.

Most treatment options include surgery and may include pre- or postoperative radiotherapy and adjuvant chemotherapy.

Surgery is often presented as the best option for a curative outcome, but it can carry with it long-term changes in lifestyle (which are not always discussed openly with patients) such as limited stomach capacity and permanently altered eating habits, or formation of a temporary or permanent stoma.

THE NURSE'S ROLE

Nurses play a key role in supporting patients and their families through the decision-making process.

From the patient's point of view there are many different nurses involved in their care. For example, a patient may typically encounter the following nurses: out-patient clinic nurses, endoscopy or X-ray department nurses, pre-admission clinic nurses, named/primary nurses in the ward, district nurses and Macmillan nurses.

It can be very confusing for patients and a lack of continuity makes for difficulties with communication and can jeopardise the understanding achieved by patients, their families and their nurses.

New nursing roles are emerging, such as nurse endoscopists and gastroenterology nurse specialists whose remit is specifically to give information and facilitate com-

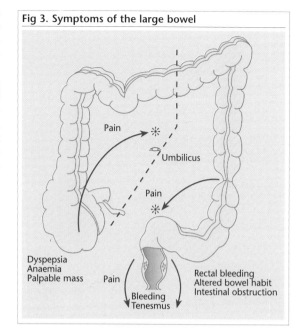

Fig 3. Symptoms of the large bowel

Pain

Umbilicus

Pain

Dyspepsia
Anaemia
Palpable mass   Pain

Bleeding
Tenesmus

Rectal bleeding
Altered bowel habit
Intestinal obstruction

munication between nurses and other members of the team caring for the patient at any given time.

Long-term support
A further feature of the nurse's role is to recognise the time period during which the patient and family are coping with the disease.

Survival figures given in Part 1, confirm that 50–60% of those with colorectal cancer will die within five years of diagnosis, and any diagnosis of cancer is for life, regardless of the time or eventual cause of death.

Thus, the disease becomes a most significant feature in the remainder of their lives. However, patients and their families learn to cope and adopt various strategies to achieve this.

However, with disjointed nursing contribution coming from different nurses at different times, evidence of their progress is at risk of being lost.

Repeated nursing assessments are carried out at different stages; for example, at the clinic when the diagnosis is made, in the ward when treatment is planned or instigated, when at home with the district nurse, and when needing palliative care with Macmillan nurse support.

Patient-held documentation, available throughout this process, would help improve both the patient's and the members of the health care teams' understanding and awareness of the individual's situation.

It would provide a vehicle for communication to which the patient, his or her family and each carer could refer, and would highlight the areas of care that the nurse should be focusing on at that moment.

Some initiatives are emerging in this area but further

work needs to be done in the patients' interests to challenge existing patterns.

HEALTH PROMOTION

Many patients actively seek to know why they have a cancer. Members of their family and friends are often anxious to know how to avoid the same fate.

In addition, the problem of digestive-tract malignancies in the UK is sufficiently frequent to warrant an increased awareness on behalf of the general public in prevention and early detection. There is a clear need for nurses to provide information regarding what steps can be taken to adopt a lifestyle which will reduce the likelihood of getting GI tract cancer.

Healthy lifestyle changes
This advice should include sensible drinking levels and the preferred types of alcohol; for example, red wine is least harmful, spirits are most harmful. It is recommended that five portions of fresh fruit and vegetables are eaten daily in combination with a low-fat diet and regular exercise provided the person being advised is able to tolerate this.

Excessive stress should be avoided in the long-term and of course everyone should be strongly advised to give up smoking. Specific advice will be required depending on the individual's need.

For example, patients with severe dysphagia should be advised on liquidised feeds in small frequent amounts, patients with colostomies will need to try foods to find out which suit them and their stoma to avoid problems with excessive flatus.

A number of written leaflets from the HEA, BACUP and other groups summarise appropriate information and could be made available to patients in support of any verbal advice given.

THINKING POINT

● Nurses are increasingly becoming involved in performing endoscopic procedures. How far do you think it is a legitimate nursing role? What attributes do nurses bring to such extended roles?

REFERENCES
1. Carper, B.A. Fundamental patterns of knowing. *Advances in Nursing Science*, 1978; 1: 13-23.
2. Office of Population and Consensus Mortality Rates Series DH2 No.19, London: HMSO, 1992.
3. Ellis, P., Cunningham, D. Management of carcinomas of the upper gastrointestinal tract. *British Medical Journal* 1994; 308: 834-838.
4. IARC. Schistosomes, liver flukes and *Heliobacter pylori*. Lyon: IARC, monograph 61, 1994.
5. Arnott, S. *Gastrointestinal cancer*. In Sikora, K., Halnan, K.E. (eds) Treatment of Cancer London: Chapman and Hall, 1990.
6. McMahon, R., Pearson, A. *Nursing as Therapy*. London: Arnold, 1991.
7. Office of Population and Census Surveys. Mortality Rates Series DH2 no.19, London: HMSO, 1992.
8. Wilson, J.M.G., Jungner, G., *Principles and Practice of Screening for Disease*. Geneva: World Health Organization,1968.

FURTHER READING
Groenwald, S.L., Frogge, M.H., Goodman, M., et al. *Part VI: The Care of Individuals with Cancer*. Boston: Jones and Bartlett, 1992.
MacLeod, M. The everyday experience of nursing practice. In: Lathlean, J., Vaughan B (eds) *Unifying Nursing Practice and Knowledge*. Oxford: Butterworth Heinnemann, 1994.
Miller, A. B. *Diet and the Aetiology of Cancer*. Heidelberg: Springer, 1989.
Speechley, V., Rosenfield, M. *Cancer Information at Your Fingertips*. London: Class, 1992.

Digestive tract cancers
Assessment

When you have read the unit and completed any further reading, you can use the questions below to test your understanding of the topic. Answers can be found on the next page

1 **Which of the more commonly occurring gastrointestinal tract cancers are the British population most likely to develop:**

1	Pancreas
2	Stomach
3	Colorectal
4	Oesophagus

2 **The first consideration in treatment for GI tract cancers is:**

1	Radiotherapy
2	Chemotherapy
3	Homeopathy
4	Surgery

3 **Laser treatment is used to:**

1	Palliate oesophageal tumours
2	Palliate rectal tumours
3	Both 1 and 2
4	Cure sigmoid tumours

4 **How many cancers occur in the digestive tract?**

1	More than half
2	About a quarter
3	2.5%
4	20%

5 **Where in the large bowel do half of all colorectal carcinomas develop?**

1	The ascending colon
2	The appendix
3	The sigmoid colon and rectum
4	The colon

6 **Life expectancy for pancreatic cancer is:**

1	Five years
2	One year
3	A normal life span, with treatment
4	Three years

7 **What investigation do patients with suspected pancreatic cancer undergo?**

1	Endoscopy
2	Colonoscopy
3	Surgery
4	ERCP

8 **Why do GI tract cancers need to be staged?**

1	To decide the most appropriate treatment
2	To find out cell type, invasion and lymph node involvement
3	Both 1 and 2
4	To predict prognosis

9 **Which organism is thought to increase the risk of stomach cancer?**

1	*Helicobacter pylori*
2	*Eschericia coli*
3	*Pseudomonas pyocyanea*
4	*Hydrochlorus gastri*

10 **Barratt's oesophagus is thought to lead to oesophageal cancer. What causes it?**

1	Excessive drinking
2	Reflux of stomach acid
3	Cell changes in the oesophageal lining
4	A high-fibre diet

11 **In which part of the world is the highest incidence of stomach cancer seen?**

1	Great Britain
2	South America
3	Eastern Europe
4	Japan and East Asia

12 **Which syndromes are likely to lead to colorectal cancer?**

1	Prader Willi
2	Lynch I and Lynch II
3	Familial polyposis coli
4	Both 2 and 3

13 **Digestive tract cancers begin to affect significant numbers of people:**

1	below 20 years
2	20-30 years
3	over 50 years
4	Normal saline

14 Familial adenomatous polyposis syndromes are called:

1	Turcot's
2	Gardner's
3	*Familial Polyposis Coli*
4	All the above

15 Patients should always be advised to :

1	Give up drinking
2	Stop smoking
3	Go back to work to distract themselves
4	Beware of diarrhoea and vomiting

16 Cancers of the liver are usually:

1	Metastatic deposits from the primary lesion in the digestive tract
2	Primary growths of the hepatic carcinoma
3	Due to malaria
4	Associated with patients who have travelled abroad recently

17 Oesophageal cancer kills how many people annually in England and Wales?

1	1:500
2	1:5000
3	1:50000
4	1:2500

ANSWERS

Digestive tract cancers

1: Which of the more commonly occurring gastrointestinal tract cancers are the British population most likely to develop:
3) Colorectal

2: The first consideration in treatment for GI tract cancers is:
4) Surgery

3: Laser treatment is used to:
1) Palliate oesophageal tumours

4: How many cancers occur in the digestive tract?
2) About a quarter

5: Where in the large bowel do half of all colorectal carcinomas develop?
3) The sigmoid colon and rectum

6: Life expectancy for pancreatic cancer is:
2) One year

7: What investigation do patients with suspected pancreatic cancer undergo?
4) ERCP

8: Why do GI tract cancers need to be staged?
8) Both 1 and 2

9: Which organism is thought to increase the risk of stomach cancer?
1) Helicobacter pylori

10: Barratt's oesophagus is thought to lead to oesophageal cancer. What causes it?
3) Cell changes in the oesophageal lining

11: In which part of the world is the highest incidence of stomach cancer seen?
4) Japan and East Asia

12: Which syndromes are likely to lead to colorectal cancer?
4) Both 2 and 3

13: Digestive tract cancers begin to affect significant numbers of people at:
3) Over 50 years

14: Familial adenomatous polyposis syndromes are called:
4) All of the above

15: Patients should always be advised to:
2) Stop smoking

16: Cancers of the liver are usually:
1) Metastatic deposits from the primary lesion in the digestive tract

17: Oesophageal cancer kills how many people annually in England and Wales?
2) 1:5000

Leukaemia
Knowledge for practice

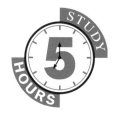

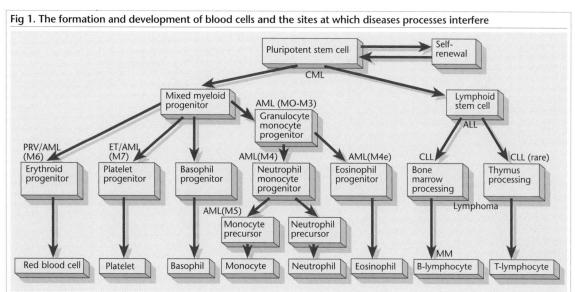

Fig 1. The formation and development of blood cells and the sites at which diseases processes interfere

The term leukaemia refers to any of a group of malignancies affecting haematological precursor cells in the bone marrow. They are characterised by the presence of large numbers of abnormal white cells in the circulating blood and reduction in the numbers of other cell types as a result of marrow displacement.

All forms of leukaemia are clonal disorders, that is to say that the malignant population all derives from a single transformed cell.

In the course of the disease further genetic changes commonly accumulate often leading to an increase in the aggressiveness of the disease.

Leukaemia is often referred to as 'cancer of the blood' but this is strictly inaccurate as the cells affected are blood-forming stem cells in the marrow. The term leukaemia derives from the Greek for 'white blood' — in cases with a very high white count a distinct layer of white blood cells can often be seen with the naked eye if a blood sample is allowed to settle out.

The bone marrow contains a small population of stem cells which is capable of both self-renewal and of producing all the different cell types found in blood. There are various stages of haematopoiesis in the course of which the capacity for cell division is gradually lost while cells acquire the capacity to carry out their specialised functions.

Leukaemia arises when cells that retain the capacity of dividing and multiplying escape from the normal control mechanisms. Fig 1 shows how different forms of leukaemia correspond to different stages of differentiation and commitment.

TYPES OF LEUKAEMIA

A basic classification of leukaemias into four categories can be made based on the progression of the untreated condition (acute or chronic) and on the cell lineage affected (lymphoid or myeloid).

The four main types (for incidence see Fig 2) are:
- Acute lymphoblastic leukaemia (ALL);
- Chronic lymphocytic leukaemia (CLL);
- Acute myeloid leukaemia (AML);
- Chronic myeloid leukaemia (CML).

The acute leukaemias are further classified according to the French American British (FAB) scheme. This subdivides acute lymphoblastic leukaemia into three subtypes (L1 to L3)[1] and acute myeloid leukaemia into eight subtypes (M0 to M7).[2]

In clinical practice leukaemia can be further defined by use of monoclonal antibodies against tissue markers.[3] This is particularly important for lymphoid malignancies, and all cases of lymphoid malignancy will be defined according to the presence of T–cell or B–cell markers.

The FAB and immunological classifications are of great importance in predicting prognosis and determining optimum therapy. The most frequent type of ALL in children is known as common ALL (cALL). This is particularly significant for prognosis.

A minority of cases of acute leukaemia remain unclassified despite application of all such techniques. Acute undifferentiated leukaemia is now a much rarer diagnosis. Some authorities consider that all cases of acute leukaemia should be assignable as either lymphoid or myeloid. Some cases of acute leukaemia have markers of both myeloid and lymphoid lineages and are classified as mixed lineage leukaemia.

It is not clear whether this is a consequence of cells of a specific lineage acquiring features of the opposite lineage or whether these are very primitive cells that are not yet committed to either lineage.

There is no classification system for CLL but there are two variant types, hairy cell leukaemia and prolymphocytic leukaemia which each account for about 10% of CLL cases. CLL is the only form for which staging is commonly used. There are several schemes of which the Rai classification is probably the most widely used.[4]

CML has a chronic phase, which typically lasts about three years but may last for decades. The disease then enters an accelerated phase which lasts for about 1.5 years. Effective treatment at this stage may return the disease to chronic phase.

Terminally, there is what is known as a blast phase, which transforms into acute leukaemia. This is usually myeloid but may be lymphoid.

PREVALENCE

Leukaemia represents about 5% of all cases of cancer, about 7000 new cases per year in the UK. The majority of leukaemia occurs in adults (about 90% of cases) and overwhelmingly in later life. In this it resembles most other forms of cancer. The one exception to this is ALL in which the peak incidence occurs between the ages of two and five years.

About 85% of cases of childhood leukaemia are ALL with almost all the remainder being acute myeloid leukaemia.

In childhood the sex ratio is approximately equal, while at all other ages there are more male cases for all types of the disease.

There is considerable variation in leukaemia incidence between ethnic groups which persists irrespective of migration and changes in life–style. An example of this is the great rarity of CLL in Asian populations. The magnitude of these variations clearly indicates genetic influences as a causative factor.

CLL is the commonest form of leukaemia with about 3500 new cases annually. There are about 600 new cases of ALL per year, about 600 of CML, and about 1900 of AML. It is quite likely that CLL, which frequently occurs as an incidental finding in an asymptomatic patient, is under-reported.

CAUSES

In most individual cases of leukaemia it is not possible to assign a specific cause. This said, there are certain clearly identified risk factors.

Radiation

Studies of Japanese A-bomb survivors and others exposed to high levels of radiation have clearly confirmed that radiation can cause leukaemia. There is, however, controversy about whether low levels of radiation are leukaemogenic.

There is a distinct cluster of childhood leukaemia in the village of Seascale, close to the Sellafield nuclear plant, for example, but there is doubt about whether the power plant is directly responsible for this.[5]

Chemical exposures

Exposure to high levels of certain chemicals has been clearly proven to be leukaemogenic. One of the best known of these chemicals is benzene which may cause myeloid leukaemia.

The most significant chemical leukaemogen in Britain is probably cigarette smoke, which has been estimated to cause as many as 25% of all cases of AML.[6] A small number of cases of AML occur as late complications of chemo and radiotherapy for cancer.

Genetic factors

The genetic implications of different incidences in different ethnic groups are borne out by the existence of certain inherited conditions that predispose to development of leukaemia.

Down's syndrome carries an approximate 20-fold increase in risk of leukaemia over background levels. Ataxia-telangiectasia, an autosomal recessive hereditary disorder characterised by cerebellar ataxia, also carries a high leukaemia risk. Although these conditions account for only a small minority of cases of leukaemia they can offer valuable insights into its aetiology.

Although leukaemia is not hereditary, there are inherited differences in susceptibility to leukaemogenic factors. There is, for example, a three-fold greater risk of CLL or related conditions in first degree relatives of patients with CLL. However, this is still a low risk and families with more than one patient are very rare.

Infection

Leukaemia is not a transmissible disease but there is at least one clearly identified human leukaemia virus. This is called the HTLV-1 and it causes a form of lymphoid leukaemia called Adult T-cell Leukaemia/Lymphoma (ATLL).

There is a theory (Greaves' hypothesis) that relates childhood ALL to patterns of exposure to infectious agents. It is proposed that in advanced societies high general standards of hygiene and small family size mean that many children have little exposure to immune stress in the first year of life.[7]

A rare consequence of delayed first immune stress is development of ALL. It is not known whether this is related to a specific infectious agent or whether it is a non-specific effect. This theory is consistent with various epidemiological findings.

CLINICAL PRESENTATION

Acute leukaemia is more likely to be symptomatic at presentation. The signs and symptoms result from accumulation of leukaemic cells in various tissues and from bone marrow overactivity and from the loss of normal blood cell production.

Marrow hyperactivity may lead to bone and joint pain, particularly in children with ALL. Some forms of acute myeloid leukaemia (AML, M4 and M5) are commonly associated with gum swelling due to accumulation of leukaemic cells. Low red cell count may lead to anaemia and fatigue, low platelets to bruising/bleeding problems and the absence of normally functional white cells predisposes to infection.

Leukaemic cells may be present in the testis or the central nervous system (CNS) with ALL. In T-cell ALL there may be a mediastinal mass made up of leukaemic cells.

Chronic leukaemia may be an incidental finding in asymptomatic patients who have had a routine blood count performed, this is particularly common in CLL.

DIAGNOSIS

Clinical features may lead to a provisional diagnosis of leukaemia. A definitive diagnosis requires demonstration of the presence of abnormal cells in the blood and/or bone marrow. Most patients will have a high or very high white cell count (that is greater than 20 x 109/l) but occasionally severe marrow damage leads to a condition known as aleukaemic leukaemia in which the white count is very low.

It may be acceptable for an older patient with CLL to be diagnosed on the basis of a blood count alone. In all other situations a bone marrow biopsy is necessary to confirm the diagnosis and to assess the degree of marrow displacement. Specific stains and the use of immunological tests allow very precise classification of leukaemia.

Cytogenetic analysis of the abnormal cells is of great value in the classification of leukaemia. The presence of a characteristic chromosome abnormality called the Philadelphia chromosome is particularly characteristic of CML. Although the diagnosis of leukaemia is usually clear-cut some infections may cause a transient leukaemia-like condition called a leukaemoid reaction. This may also be seen in infants with Down's syndrome.

Most cases of leukaemoid reaction can be distinguished on the basis a test called the neutrophil alkaline phosphatase score. Alkaline phosphatase is an enzyme which is present at high levels in leukaemoid reactions but is low in leukaemic cells. The other key distinguishing feature is the absence of significant chromosome abnormalities in leukaemoid reactions.

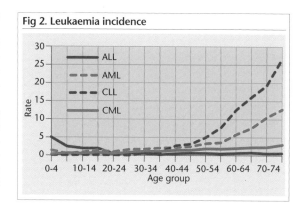

Fig 2. Leukaemia incidence

TREATMENT

The mainstay of leukaemia treatment is chemotherapy. In children with ALL prophylactic radiotherapy may be administered to prevent testicular or CNS recurrence. Either allo- or autograft bone marrow transplantation may be offered depending on the form of the disease.

The high procedure-related mortality in older patients (over about 55 years) needs to be taken into account in allogeneic transplantation.

Acute leukaemia
Acute leukaemia, particularly in younger patients, may be curable with high-dose chemotherapy. In children with ALL the cure rate may be as high as 75%.[8] In light of the high success rate with chemotherapy in children bone marrow transplant is only considered for children, with features of poor-risk disease or who have relapsed on treatment.

Among the features predictive of poor response to standard therapy are: aged under two and over 10 years; very high initial white count; all types of leukaemia other than cALL; male sex and black ethnic origin.

The success rate of chemotherapy for children with AML is poor largely because of the development of drug resistance. Adults with ALL frequently respond well initially but here again the problem of drug resistance leads to a comparatively poor overall prognosis.

Adult AML can be classified on the basis of laboratory findings as good risk, standard risk or high risk. Patients with good-risk disease tend to respond very well to chemotherapy.

Patients with poor-risk disease will respond poorly to chemotherapy and are candidates for early allogeneic bone marrow transplant if a donor is available. The selection of treatment for standard-risk patients may be problematic and it is this group in which good controlled trials may be of most value.

Chronic leukaemia

CML is generally considered to be treatable but not curable with chemotherapy. The only treatment considered curative is successful allogeneic bone marrow transplantation. Autologous bone marrow or all peripheral blood stem cell transplant may return CML from accelerated phase to chronic phase.

In many patients with CLL, treatment is unnecessary, at least initially. This is because the natural history of the disease is indolent. When treatment of older patients is considered desirable this is usually with oral chemotherapy as an outpatient. Younger patients may be considered for a potentially curative allogeneic bone marrow transplant.

The side-effects of treatment are essentially those of all forms of anticancer treatment. In the short term these are the consequences of damage to healthy dividing cells such as neutropenia, hair loss and gastrointestinal disturbances. In the longer term, infertility may prove distressing for younger patients.

There is clear evidence that patients who retain their fertility despite having received chemotherapy or radiotherapy are at no increased risk of having abnormal offspring. Children who have received prophylactic treatment against CNS recurrence may experience educational problems. These are not usually very severe although there will be a clearly detectable reduction in IQ.

THINKING POINT

● How far should nurses influence debates about possible environmental influences on health, such as nuclear power plants?

PART TWO

The role of the nurse

The diagnosis and treatment of leukaemia have a profound effect on the patient. People diagnosed with acute forms of the disease will usually be young and previously fit and although people who develop chronic leukaemia will be older, anyone who learns they have the disease will experience a radical change in their lifestyle both because of the disease and the side effects of its treatment.

Treatment for AML initially takes the form of high dose chemotherapy over a short period. Treatment for ALL is spread over a longer period. Treatment is followed by supportive therapy consisting of blood product transfusions and antibiotics to prevent bacterial, fungal and viral infections.

Nurses, regardless of the setting in which they work, play an important part in helping people with leukaemia deal with the limitations placed on them by the disease. The information in this book is designed for the non-specialist nurse who encounters people with leukaemia infrequently. It outlines the major areas of nursing care required in terms of guarding against the risks of infection and bleeding and dealing with the debilitating effects of the disease and its treatment. The nursing issues discussed deal principally with symptoms and treatment for the person with a diagnosis of acute leukaemia.

Whichever form of the disease is diagnosed, the patient will have to deal with the symptoms over a long period. Nursing care may at times have to compensate for what

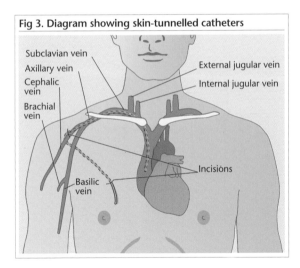

Fig 3. Diagram showing skin-tunnelled catheters

Subclavian vein
Axillary vein
Cephalic vein
Brachial vein
Basilic vein
External jugular vein
Internal jugular vein
Incisions

people cannot do for themselves. However, care should aim to help the person adapt and maintain their independence. This requires a facilitative approach that takes its lead from what the patient is experiencing.

THE RISK OF INFECTION

In leukaemia, white cells that usually provide defence against infection are unable to fulfil their normal function because they are immature and proliferate in the bone marrow, which leads to a reduced production of red cells and platelets.

The immature white cells do not function normally, placing the patient at risk of potentially life-threatening infection, the commonest cause of death in this patient group.[9] As the disease progresses the neutrophil count falls further giving rise to the state known as neutropenia.

Certain types of cytotoxic chemotherapy also affect the bone marrow, suppressing not only the production of white cells but also platelets and red blood cells.

Common infections in leukaemia patients are endogenous bacterial infections caused by pseudomonas, *Escherichia coli* and klebsiella from the gut, and exogenous infections caused by *Staphylococcus aureus* around intravenous catheter sites. *Staphylococcus epidermidis* from the skin can also infect the sites of central venous catheters.

A person with leukaemia is at particular risk of stomatitis because of both the disease process and chemotherapy. Chemotherapy affects cell division, and cells in the mouth normally divide quickly to maintain the integrity of the mouth.

Chemotherapy interferes with this process and the mucous membranes become fragile and prone to infection. Fungal infections of the mouth are mainly caused by *Candida albicans*. Fungal infections in the lungs are caused either by candida or aspergillous present in dust.

The measures to minimise risk can be divided into monitoring and preventive measures.

Monitoring
Neutropenic patients are not able to respond to infection and, in the absence of white cells, the normal signs of infection such as inflammation may not be present. Pyrexia, however, will be present (>38°C). Regular monitoring,

and teaching patients and their families to watch for signs of infection, is therefore central to nursing care.

In addition to the normal measures to observe for infection, such as monitoring vital signs, extra attention must be paid to other signs such as sore throats, rigor, cough, burning on micturition, shortness of breath, and diarrhoea.

Mucous membranes are prone to damage and the mouth is particularly vulnerable. Inflammation may be indicated by a burning feeling in the mouth as well as obvious lesions such as those associated with Herpes zoster. Local or systemic analgesia will be required. The skin-tunnelled catheter used for administering chemotherapy and supportive treatment is also a potential source of systemic infection and must be closely observed for inflammation and/or discharge.

If infection is suspected, the source must be isolated and blood, urine, sputum, swabs of any wounds or catheter sites, and stool samples should be obtained for microbiological examination. A chest X-ray will also be required if a chest infection is suspected.

Preventive measures
Because of the fragility of the mucous membranes, mouth care is very important and should take place after every meal. Patients should be advised to buy a small headed toothbrush with soft bristles and to use short horizontal strokes when brushing to avoid contact with the gums. Chlorhexidine mouthwash is used for its antibacterial properties and nystatin suspension as a prophylactic against *C. albicans*.

Food is a potential source of infection in a neutropenic patient and the need for a nutritious diet must be balanced against minimising bacteria in food.

A low microbial diet (Table 1) is essential to prevent

Table 1. Low microbial diet		
Item	*Allowed*	*Not allowed*
Soup	Hot soup, tinned or home-made	Cold fresh soup
Meat, fish and poultry	Well cooked (before expiry date), tinned	Raw, cold non-cooked
Take-aways	None	All take-aways
Cheese	Pasteurised cheese including cottage cheese	Non-pasteurised (eg, Brie)
Eggs	Well cooked eggs only; eg, hard boiled or omelette	Raw
Bread	Any fresh bread	
Vegetables	Any cooked	Raw, for example salads
Fruit	Fresh fruit that is easily peeled and undamaged	Unpeeled fruit
Desserts	Cooked puddings, jelly, ice cream	
Drinks	Virtually all drinks	
Others	Sweets, salt, chocolate, pickles, pasteurised yoghurt, packet soups, pot noodle, pre-prepared meals from major supermarket chains	Pepper, fresh mayonnaise

LEUKAEMIA

gastro-intestinal infections. Uncooked foods and unpasteurised dairy products should be avoided. Take-away foods are definitely off the menu as they may be reheated and so carry a risk of bacterial contamination.

Diet is also important from the point of view of avoiding constipation.

During treatment the mucous membranes of the rectum are also prone to becoming friable and constipation can cause trauma, bleeding and infection. Enemas and suppositories must be avoided and constipation should be prevented through diet, good fluid intake and aperients as needed.

Infections of the respiratory tract can be minimised through avoiding contact with people with colds or flu. Other communicable infections are potentially life-threatening so it is vital to avoid people who have or who have been in contact with chicken pox, measles or herpes.

The extent to which people should be isolated is open to debate. In hospital, a single room is desirable, although the effectiveness of single rooms for strict protective isolation has been questioned.[10] Anyone in contact with patients should wash their hands with an antimicrobial agent, dry them thoroughly and wear a plastic apron. Wrist watches must be removed.

The room should be kept clean and sources of bacteria such as standing water, flowers and fresh fruit should be avoided while the person is neutropenic. Essential equipment, such as thermometers and sphygmomanometers, should be kept in the room for use with one patient at a time. Bed linen must be changed daily.

Good personal hygiene is essential. Commensal bacteria can cause disease while the white cell count is low. A daily bath or shower helps minimise the risk of infection.

At discharge it is important that the patient and their family are familiar with the principles involved in avoiding infection.

They will need to respond quickly to infection if it occurs at home and apply preventive measures as part of a daily routine.

The immune system can take up to six months to recover fully following high-dose chemotherapy and bone marrow transplantation.

THE SKIN-TUNNELLED CATHETER

Skin-tunnelled catheters (STCs), for example Hickman–Broviac lines, may be used to provide long-term venous access to the patient's circulatory system making the administration of drugs (chemotherapy and antibiotics), blood products and fluids less traumatic, as well as providing easy access for taking blood samples and haemodynamic monitoring.

They are usually inserted via the subclavian vein and tunnelled subcutaneously to appear between the sternum and the nipple, either under general or local anaesthetic (Fig 3).

These catheters have an antimicrobial cuff on the subcutaneous segment. This causes a local inflammatory reaction causing fixation and a barrier to infection in about one to two weeks.

STCs can remain in place for several months with appropriate management.

STCs require regular dressing changes. Frequency of dressings depends on the product used. They also need flushing every other day. Ultimately, this will usually be done by the patient and/or his or her carer. Both procedures must be performed aseptically. Entry sites should not be immersed in the bath and should be protected in the shower. After exit sutures are removed (day 21) no dressing is usually required.[11]

SUPPORTING THE PATIENT

The speed at which people come to terms with caring for their STC varies. The aim is to give patient and carer the knowledge and skills needed to care for the STC independently.

STC insertion takes place soon after diagnosis at a time when the patient is coming to terms with a life–threatening illness.

Its management requires reasonable dexterity and involves considerable risks, such as infection, blockage, air embolism and splits in the line. It is a constant reminder to patients of their ill health.

Preparing the patient to care for the STC should be guided by their reaction to it and their own willingness to take over its care.

Teaching should be based on a thorough assessment of the patient, their family, home life and how they are adapting to diagnosis. It should proceed at a pace dictated by the patient's own needs. Ultimately the patient will ideally be in a position to clean the catheter site aseptically and change the dressing daily following their bath or shower and flush the line twice a week when not in use.

THROMBOCYTOPAENIA

Uncontrolled bleeding is the second highest cause of mortality in people with leukaemia. The proliferation of immature white blood cells reduces the production of erythrocytes and platelets, and chemotherapy also reduces the platelet count. Consequently, patients are prone to bleeding caused by relatively minor trauma. Once again, nursing intervention can be characterised in terms of monitoring and prevention.

Monitoring
Vital signs should be monitored for signs of blood loss. Apart from tachycardia and hypotension, blood loss may be detected by observing the gums and other mucous membranes. Nurses should also be alert to conjunctival haemorrhage, haematemesis, haematuria, melaena, changes in conscious state — suggesting intracranial bleeding — or increased girth — suggesting abdominal bleeding.

Prevention

A wide range of every day and clinical activities are limited by the risk of bleeding. To some extent these can be predicted by the platelet count, where a count of less than 10 000/mm^3 indicates a risk of bleeding for the apyrexial patient, while a count of 100 000/mm^3 or more indicates little or no risk.

Procedures to be avoided include: intramuscular and subcutaneous injection, the use of intravenous cannulae, taking temperatures rectally, use of enemas and suppositories and urinary catheterisation, although this is not always clinically possible. Patients should be advised to take the following measures:
● Use an electric razor if shaving is necessary;
● Avoid using a hard toothbrush or dental floss;
● Avoid blowing the nose too hard;
● Watch for blood in bowel movements, vomit or sputum;
● Report headaches;
● Avoid restrictive and tight clothes.

If the patient needs help to move this should be given with great care to avoid bruising. If bleeding or trauma occur, prompt action is needed to limit bleeding. Direct pressure should be applied to any puncture site for three–to–five minutes. Menstruation is inhibited by administration of noresthisterone 5–10mg, three times a day.

Platelet transfusion

The presence of mucosal bleeding or purpura in a patient with a low platelet count indicates the need for platelet transfusion. However, platelets are often given prophylactically to maintain the count with an alternate daily transfusion often sufficient.[10]

Platelet transfusions are generally given over 20–30 minutes per unit, with three to five units being administered at one infusion.

As with transfusions of whole blood there is a risk of allergic reaction. A steroid and antihistamine may be administered prophylactically in anticipation of this. A platelet filter may also be used to prevent alloimmunisation.

ANAEMIA

Anaemia can be present at diagnosis as a result of the disease or may occur as a consequence of treatment. The patient may experience lethargy, fatigue, shortness of breath or pallor. Anaemia is treated with red cell (blood) transfusions.

One unit of packed cells is transfused to replace one gram of haemoglobin. Each unit is infused over three or four hours. Hourly observations are essential to recognise adverse reactions. A blood filter, steroids and an antihistamine may be prescribed with the transfusion to minimise reactions, which are common with repeated blood and platelet transfusions.

CHEMOTHERAPY

By its very nature, chemotherapy has a profound effect on normal cell function. A current trend in the treatment of acute leukaemia is to use high-dose chemotherapy, which destroys the tumour cells in the diseased bone marrow. It also suppresses the development of mature white cells, red cells and platelets, exacerbating the risk of infection and predisposition to bleeding. Chemotherapy has a range of other side-effects. Nausea and vomiting are common. Severity varies with different types of chemotherapy and anti-emetics are prescribed accordingly.

Short-term alopecia is also frequent and affects the eyebrows, eyelashes, axilla and the pubic area as well as the scalp. Regrowth starts five to eight weeks after treatment finishes. Wigs, hats or scarves can be used, according to preference.

High-dose chemotherapy may cause infertility, especially in men, and sperm banking may be considered. In women, the situation is more complex but some evaluation of fertility can be made on the basis of menstrual cycle and blood chemistry.

Chemotherapy does not necessarily end any chance of having children but it is an issue that should be discussed before treatment starts.

Sexual activity may become more difficult. As well as the fatigue and anxiety that may diminish sexual drive, chemotherapy makes genital mucous membranes more fragile, predisposing to infections or bleeding. Nurses may need to provide advice and support on this subject.

PSYCHOLOGICAL EFFECTS

Leukaemia has a profound effect on people. Acute leukaemias in particular confront previously young, fit people with the threat of death and the certainty of treatment that will have a profound effect on them and their families. The cumulative physical and psychological effects of both the disease and its treatment cause tremendous fatigue.

Patients and their families may experience anxiety, denial, panic, anger, relief, depression, fear, sexual problems, financial difficulties and problems with relationships. Working through these feelings is important if psychological healing is to take place. Patients and carers may need the support of a professional counsellor or Macmillan nurse. The fear of relapse is constant even years after treatment and some form of long–term psychological support may be needed

THINKING POINT

● The physical effects of leukaemia will probably mean that the patient's ability to take in information is impaired. What strategies can you use to promote understanding of and access to relevant and useful information?

PART THREE

Advances in treatment

From 1950 to 1985 the percentage of children newly diagnosed with ALL who enjoyed a 10–year remission rose from less than 5% to 60%. Since then the rate has continued to improve, although more slowly.[12]

The survival rates for other forms of leukaemia and other groups of patients have also improved significantly, although less dramatically. Even where improvements in overall survival have changed least, patients' quality of life has been greatly improved.

DEVELOPMENT OF LEUKAEMIA TREATMENT

The most important development in therapy for leukaemia was the introduction of chemotherapy. This began as early as 1948 with a drug called aminopterin. Other drugs were shown to be effective. The results of chemotherapy were initially quite dramatic but sadly it was found that, although many patients achieved an initial complete remission, in most cases this was of limited duration.

When patients relapsed, their treatment was switched to another drug, following the pattern of treatment for an antibiotic–resistant infection. Such sequential therapy often significantly prolonged life but eventually the disease failed to respond to any therapy. A major problem was a tendency for a form of multidrug resistance to develop to all forms of chemotherapy. At this time, delaying the inevitability of death was thought to be the best that could be achieved.

In the mid-1960s, multidrug chemotherapy was proposed whereby a patient was treated according to a protocol consisting of several drugs in combination.

This approach was found to be far more effective than allowing resistance to develop, and by the beginning of the 1970s, the cure of a significant percentage of children with ALL was considered achievable.[12]

Cure rates were improved still further by the addition of further blocks of treatment to consolidate remission, and current clinical trials are seeking to establish the optimal number of blocks of consolidation.

THE CENTRAL NERVOUS SYSTEM

A further key element in treatment of childhood ALL was the introduction of prophylactic treatment to the central nervous system to reduce the risk of relapse.

The CNS is a 'sanctuary site' because there are normally small numbers of lymphocytes present and the blood-brain barrier blocks the entry of drugs into the cerebrospinal fluid.

This means that it is possible for leukaemic cells to survive here, leading to meningeal relapse. This is a significant problem in both adults and children if CNS prophy-

laxis is not given. One of the few instances in which radiotherapy is used in treatment of leukaemia is in prophylactic treatment of CNS (cranial irradiation).

The methods available to prevent relapse in the CNS are cranial irradiation, injection of methotrexate into the cerebro-spinal fluid by lumbar puncture (intrathecal methotrexate) or high–dose intravenous methotrexate (to raise the blood concentration and overcome the blood-brain barrier).

When a combination of cranial irradiation and intrathecal methotrexate are used together, the side-effects may be significant and there is particular concern about possible intellectual impairment secondary to cranial irradiation. There are currently trials to establish whether intrathecal methotrexate (alone or with high-dose intravenous methotrexate) can remove the need for cranial irradiation.

TESTICULAR RELAPSE

Isolated testicular relapse does not appear to be a problem with adults but is seen in children. It is usually relatively easy to overcome isolated testicular relapse and for this reason testicular prophylaxis is not routinely given. This is the only other site in which relapse outside the marrow is at all common.

Since 1970 the aims have been to improve the success rate and reduce long-term side-effects in treatment of childhood leukaemia and to achieve cure rates in adult patients approaching those for childhood leukaemia.

ACUTE LEUKAEMIAS

Many of the drugs used in cancer chemotherapy are cell-cycle-specific — they are only able to kill cells that are actively dividing. In acute leukaemia, a high proportion of the tumour population will be susceptible at any given time. For this reason, acute leukaemia is usually responsive to chemotherapy and most patients will achieve remission when initially treated.

By giving chemotherapy in a series of blocks with 'rest' periods, the damage to healthy cells can be minimised and the tumour cell kill maximised. Those tumour cells that were resting at the time of one block are likely to have started to divide, and so be susceptible to chemotherapy by the next scheduled treatment block. It is possible to achieve long-lasting disease-free remission in acute leukaemia with chemotherapy alone. Obstacles to treatment in acute leukaemia relate to the possibility of multidrug resistance, and a key area of research is the development of new approaches to overcome this problem.

The most common mechanism of resistance to chemotherapy is through increased production of proteins in the cell membrane which remove toxins, including therapeutic drugs, from the cell. Extensive laboratory

Table 2. Poor prognostic features in acute lymphoblastic leukaemia

Feature	Poor risk	Good risk
Age	<2 years or >10 years	Age 2–10
Sex	Male	Female
Ethnic origin	Black	Caucasian
Initial white blood cell count	>20 x 10^9/l at presentation	<20 x 10^9/l at presentation
Immunological subtype	T-cell or, to a lesser extent, null cell disease	Common ALL
French American British sub-type	L3 (Burkitt's-like ALL)	L1 or L2
Cytogenetics	Presence of Philadelphia chromosone	High hyperdiploid (large number of extra chromosones)

research is being carried out in a number of centres into possible ways of blocking these proteins from exporting drugs.[13] This may be achievable by a non-specific blocking of the protein's functions or more selectively by modifying the drugs to overcome this mechanism of resistance.

Acute lymphoblastic leukaemia

Most children with ALL respond well to combination chemotherapy. About a third will either show a poorer initial response, possibly failing to enter remission, or will develop multidrug resistance. In many cases this can be predicted on the basis of either patient characteristics or presenting features of the disease.

One group of patients does not have the typical features of poor–risk ALL but nonetheless show resistance to standard regimens. In order to ensure that a significant minority of patients are not undertreated, most children with ALL are probably overtreated. This means that if it were possible to predict which children will respond well to treatment, it would in turn be possible to reduce the intensity of treatment, and thus of side–effects, for those children.14 It would also be valuable to predict which children could safely omit the prophylactic treatment to the CNS and testis, and be spared those associated side-effects.

The Leukaemia Research Fund ALL cytogenetics database at the Royal Free Hospital, London, is attempting to achieve just such predictions. The key is study of the exact chromosome changes present in the leukaemic cells. These chromosome abnormalities are not inherited but, as can be shown by their absence in other body cells, are an intrinsic part of the disease.

Although the exact pattern varies from patient to patient there are certain features that are consistently associated with good–risk disease, while others are predictors of poor response to standard therapy. By correlating the chromosome changes with the presenting clinical data and the clinical progress of the patient, the ALL database is bringing us nearer the time when each child will receive treatment tailored to their predicted sensitivity to treatment. The goal is that no child should suffer either a relapse as a consequence of undertreatment or avoidable side–effects due to overtreatment.

Although all newly diagnosed patients are included in the database, most adults present with poor-risk disease (specifically the presence of the Philadelphia chromosome), which means the work of the database is likely to offer most benefits to children.

In both high-risk children and adult patients the introduction of bone marrow or peripheral blood stem cell transplant in first remission has greatly improved prospects for survival. Some authorities have argued that bone marrow transplant can be reserved for second remission and used only if the patient relapses.[14]

Acute myeloid leukaemia

Most patients with AML will achieve initial remission. A high proportion will relapse and go on to develop multidrug resistance (Table 2). On the basis of various risk factors, particularly cytogenetics, it is possible to divide AML into three categories — poor risk (35%), standard risk (41%) and good risk (24%).[15] Most patients with good–risk disease will respond well to chemotherapy and have a good chance of achieving long–term disease–free remission with chemotherapy alone. Poor-risk patients have very little chance of long-term survival from chemotherapy and, if a suitable donor is available, should be considered for a bone marrow or peripheral blood stem cell transplant in first complete remission.[16]

The most problematic group is the 41% with standard-risk disease, and a current clinical trial is attempting to determine what should be the role, if any, of bone marrow transplant in this group. It may be that a more extensive study of the correlation between cytogenetics and treatment outcome in this group would be of value.

Many patients with acute leukaemia are over the age of 55, which is the current cut-off point for consideration of bone marrow or peripheral blood stem cell transplant at most centres. Some of these patients may be able to benefit from autologous transplants but this still only applies to a minority.

A particular form of AML (FAB subtype M3 — acute promyelocytic leukaemia) has been found to respond well to a derivative of vitamin A called retinoic acid. This is a relatively new drug belonging to a group called differentiation agents. These drugs induce the leukaemic cells to mature into end-stage cells and eventually to undergo programmed cell death (apoptosis). If retinoic acid is given alone, the patients will eventually relapse, but this can be prevented by use of consolidation chemotherapy with standard agents. The introduction of retinoic acid is of particular importance because patients with M3 AML who have conventional drugs for remission induction are at great risk of catastrophic haemorrhage. Their leukaemic cells contain granules that release coagulation-inducing factors and cause massive disseminated intravascular coagulation followed by lethal haemorrhaging.

CHRONIC LEUKAEMIA

In patients with chronic leukaemia very few of the tumour cells will be actively dividing at any given time.

This means that drugs that act only against dividing cells will kill a much smaller percentage of the tumour cell population in chronic leukaemia than in acute leukaemia. The benefit of using cell-cycle-specific agents is that they have minimal toxicity to non-dividing normal cells — only those tissues with very active cell turnover are vulnerable.

Even with these agents the therapeutic dose range between ineffectively low dosages and unacceptably toxic levels is very narrow. In chronic leukaemia, it is necessary to combine use of cell-cycle-specific and non cell-cycle-specific agents.

Chronic leukaemias are generally considered incurable by chemotherapy. There is evidence that some very tissue-specific agents used against CLL may offer the possibility of cure.[17] These agents are relatively new, however, and it is not yet clear whether they will prove curative.

Chronic lymphocytic leukaemia
A high proportion of patients with CLL present at an advanced age with a slowly developing condition. These patients will require either no specific therapy or only oral low-dose chemotherapy.

A small number of younger patients present with the condition. For these patients such an approach would be unacceptable. For this minority of patients a new group of drugs, the purine analogues, is offering promising results. These drugs, which block DNA synthesis, appear to be selectively active against the lymphoid cells, which is a great benefit.

The key drugs in this group are 2-CDA and fludarabine and both have been used in CLL.[18] A welcome feature of these drugs is their efficacy in previously heavily treated patients.

With increasing experience in the use of these drugs and in their side-effects, they may be used more widely with older patients who currently would not otherwise receive curative therapy.

Younger patients with CLL may be candidates for bone marrow transplant. There is clear evidence that allogeneic transplants may offer the chance of cure.[18] A distinct subtype of CLL called hairy cell leukaemia tends to affect a younger population. This form of the disease is responsive to interferon and good results had been achieved with this biological agent.[19] The purine analogues have been found to be extremely effective in hairy cell leukaemia with some patients apparently achieving cure with a single course of treatment.

Chronic myeloid leukaemia
CML typically shows three distinct phases: a chronic phase in which the disease progresses slowly; an accelerated phase in which the condition becomes more aggressive; and a terminal blast phase, which may be lymphoid or myeloid.

CML is treatable with chemotherapy but the only curative option is generally considered to be a successful allogeneic bone marrow or peripheral blood stem cell transplant.

An autologous transplant of marrow or peripheral blood stem cells obtained during chronic phase and re-infused in accelerated phase may be effective in achieving a reversion to chronic phase. Allogeneic transplant has poor outcomes in older people and for many a matched donor cannot be found.

One of the hallmarks of CML is the presence of the Philadelphia chromosome. It results from the exchange of small pieces of chromosomes 9 and 22 which is noted as t(9;22) or Ph1. This feature is so consistent that it has been suggested that so-called Ph1-negative CML, is not true CML, but a different form of leukaemia altogether. The Ph1 chromosome contains an abnormal gene called BCR/ABL, which is made up of two genes normally on different chromosomes. This gene produces a protein known to be directly involved in the pathology of CML.

A new approach to the treatment of CML, and potentially of other cancers, is the production of an artificial section of DNA called antisense DNA, which will bind to the BCR/ABL gene and block production of its harmful protein.

This technique has been shown to work in the laboratory but there are problems in transferring it to clinical use. A closely related approach is the use of the abnormal section of DNA as a DNA vaccine to attempt to induce an immune response that will be specific to the leukaemia cell. Attempts to induce cancer-specific immune reactions in a more conventional way have failed.

A completely new approach to therapy is the use of the

immune system as a channel to deliver cytotoxic drugs directly and specifically to the tumour cells. This is known as immunotherapy and again offers the prospect of effectiveness against a range of cancers currently refractory to treatment.[20] It relies on generating monoclonal antibodies that will target tumour cells very precisely. These antibodies are bonded to cytotoxic agents, which can be released within the tumour cell, achieving a high tumour cell kill with few or no side-effects.

THINKING POINTS

● What are the likely tensions between the needs of the hospital, such as diagnosis and treatment, and the patient's needs? How can nurses help reconcile these?

● A patient's family want to be with him or her all the time to provide care. How would you go about supporting this while ensuring family members get adequate rest?

REFERENCES
1. Bennett, J.M., Catovsky, D., Daniel, M.T. et al and The French-American-British Cooperative Group. The morphologic classification of acute lymphocytic leukaemia: Concordance among observers and clinical correlations. *British Journal of Haematology* 1981; **47**: 553-561.
2. Bennett, J.M. Catovsky, D., Daniel, M.T. et al. Proposed revised criteria for the classification of acute myeloid leukaemia. *Annals of Internal Medicine* 1985; **103**: 6230-6235.
3. Campbell, K. Understanding acute and chronic myeloid leukaemia. *Nursing Times* 1995; **91**: 47. 36-38.
4. Rai, K.R. A Critical Analysis of Staging in CLL. *Chronic Lymphocytic Leukaemia: Recent Progress and Future Direction.* New York: Alan R. Liss, 1987.
5. Draper, G.I., Stiller, C.A., Cartwright, R.A. et al. Cancer in Cumbria and in the vicinity of Sellafield nuclear installation, 1963-90. *British Journal of Medicine* 1993; **306**: 89-94.
6. Cartwright, R.A. *Epidemiology: Leukaemia.* Oxford: Blackwell, 1992.
7. Greaves, M.F. *Etiology of childhood acute lymphoblastic leukaemia: A soluble problem? Acute Leukaemia: UCLA Symposium on Molecular and Cellular Biology.* New York: Academic Press, 1989.
8. Childhood ALL Collaborative Group. Duration and intensity of maintenance chemotherapy in acute lymphoblastic leukaemia: overview of 42 trials involving 12 000 randomised children. *Lancet* 1996; **347**: 9018, 1783-1788.
9. Porter, H.J. Caring for autologous transplant patients in an open ward environment. *Bone Marrow Transplant* 1995; **15**: supp 2, S197.
10. Ruffell, J.A., Poon, M-C., Jones, A.R. et al. Allogenic bone marrow transplantation without protective isolation in adults with malignant disease. *Lancet* 1992; **339**: 38.
11. Mallett, J., Bailey, C. (eds). *The Royal Marsden NHS Trust Manual of Clinical Nursing Procedure.* London: Blackwell Science, 1996.
12. Lilleyman, J.S. *Childhood Leukaemia: The Facts.* Oxford: Oxford University Press, 1994.
13. Michieli, M., Giacca, M., Fanin, R. et al. Mdr-1 gene amplification in acute lymphoblastic leukaemia prior to antileukaemic treatment. *British Journal of Haematology* 1991; **78**: 288.
14. Hughes-Jones, N.C., Wickramasinghe, S.N. *Lecture Notes on Haematology.* Oxford: Blackwell Science, 1996.
15. WWW document. Estey, E.H. (1996) The role of cytogenetics in the treatment of AML. URL http//www.meds.com/mol/leukemia/curr1.html
16. Tallman, M.S., Kopecky, K.J., Amos, D. et al. Analysis of prognostic factors for the outcome of marrow transplantation or further chemotherapy for patients with acute non-lymphocytic leukaemia in first remission. *Journal of Clinical Oncology* 1989; **7**: 326-337.
17. WWW document. O'Brien, M.E.R., Catovsky, D. (1996) Fludarabine in lymphoproliferative disorders: an active new drug. URL http://www.leukemia.demon.co.uk/purine1/htm
18. Keating, M.J. Chronic lymphocytic leukaemia. In: Henderson, E.S., Lister, T.A., Greaves, M.F. (eds). *Leukaemia.* Philadelphia: Saunders, 1996.
19. Hoffman, M., Rai, K. Hairy cell leukaemia. In: Henderson, E.S., Lister, T.A., Greaves, M.F. (eds). *Leukaemia.* Philadelphia: Saunders, 1996.
20. Perentesis, J.P., Kersey, J.H. Biologic therapy of leukaemia. In: Henderson, E.S., Lister, T.A., Greaves, M.F. (eds). *Leukaemia.* Philadelphia: Saunders, 1996.

Useful address

Leukaemia Research Fund, 43 Great Ormond Street, London, WC1N 3JJ. Tel: 0171-405 0101.

LEUKAEMIA

Leukaemia

Assessment

When you have read the unit and completed any further reading, you can use the questions below to test your understanding of the topic. Answers can be found on the next page

1 **Bone marrow stem cells are capable of :**

1	Production of mature blood cells
2	Self-renewal
3	Both of the above
4	Neither of the above

2 **Which one of the following is not one of the main types of leukaemia:**

1	Chronic lymphocytic leukaemia
2	Acute myeloid leukaemia
3	Hodgkin's disease
4	Lymphoma

3 **Hairy cell leukaemia is a form of:**

1	Acute lymphoblastic leukaemia
2	Chronic lymphocytic leukaemia
3	Acute myeloid leukaemia
4	Chronic myeloid leukaemia

4 **Leukaemia represents what percentage of all cases of cancer:**

1	5%
2	25%
3	50%
4	2.5%

5 **The most common form of leukaemia in children is:**

1	Acute myeloid leukaemia
2	Chronic myeloid leukaemia
3	Acute lymphoblastic leukaemia
4	Chronic lymphocytic leukaemia

6 **Most forms of leukaemia are:**

1	More common in females than males
2	More common in males than females
3	Equally common in females and males
4	Commoner among the under-5s

7 **Which of the following conditions is not associated with an increased risk of leukaemia:**

1	Down's Syndrome
2	Ataxia-telangiectasia
3	Sickle cell disease
4	None of the above

8 **Combination chemotherapy means:**

1	The use of chemotherapy in combination with radiotherapy
2	The use of a combination of drugs in the course of chemotherapy
3	The use of different chemotherapy drugs in sequence, changing the drug in use as resistance rises
4	The use of both bone marrow transplant and chemotherapy

9 **Chemotherapy used alone has a significant chance of curing:**

1	Chronic leukaemia but not acute leukaemia
2	Acute leukaemia but not chronic leukaemia
3	Both acute and chronic leukaemia
4	No cure has yet been found, although remission has become more common and lasts longer

10 **Neutropenia means:**

1	A raised white blood count
2	A raised neutrophil count
3	A reduced neutrophil count
4	None of the above

11 **Thrombocytopenia means:**

1	Reduced levels of thrombi
2	A reduction of platelets
3	A raised level of platelets
4	Lack of enzyme needed for clotting

12 **The aim of care in the patient who is neutropenic is:**

1	To offer the patient optimal protection from infections
2	Prompt recognition and treatment when infections do occur
3	To reinforce the need for strict personal hygiene
4	All of the above

LEUKAEMIA

13 **The aim of care in the patient with thrombocytopenia is:**

- 1 To recognise signs of bleeding
- 2 To prevent bleeding
- 3 Both of the above
- 4 None of the above

14 **A low microbial diet is essential for the following reason:**

- 1 It provides a strict dietary regime
- 2 It prevents enteric infections
- 3 Macrobiotic diets are useful in patients with cancer
- 4 It prevents constipation

15 **Invasive procedures such as intramuscular or subcutaneous injections, suppositories or catheterisation must be avoided in the patient who is neutropenic and thrombocytopenic**

for the following reason:

- 1 In order to avoid trauma
- 2 Because they predispose to bleeding
- 3 Because they increase risks of infection
- 4 All the above

16 **A skin-tunnelled catheter is used for:**

- 1 Venous access
- 2 Administration of intravenous therapy
- 3 Transfusing blood products
- 4 All the above

17 **Good personal hygiene on the part of the patient is important because:**

- 1 It gives the patient something to do
- 2 It reduces the risk of commensal infection
- 3 It prevents the spread of the MRSA infection
- 4 It maintains patient dignity

ANSWERS

Leukaemia

1: Bone marrow stem cells are capable of:
3) Both of the above

2: Which one of the following is not one of the main types of leukaemia:
3) Hodgkin's disease

3: Hairy cell leukaemia is a form of:
2) Chronic lymphocytic leukaemia

4: Leukaemia represents what percentage of all cases of cancer:
1) 5%

5: The most common form of leukaemia in children is:
3) Acute lymphoblastic leukaemia

6: Most forms of leukaemia are:
2) More common in males than females

7: Which of the following conditions is not associated with an increased risk of leukaemia?
3) Sickle cell disease

8: Combination chemotherapy means:
2) Use of a combination of drugs in the course of chemotherapy

9: Chemotherapy used alone has a significant chance of curing:
4) No cure has yet been found although remission has become

more common and lasts longer

10: Neutropenia means:
3) A reduced neutrophil count

11: Thrombocytopenia means:
2) A reduction of platelets

12: The aim of care in the patient who is neutropenic is:
4) All of the above

13: The aim of care in the patient with thrombocytopenia is:
3) Both of the above

14: A low microbial diet is essential for the following reason:
2) It prevents potential enteric infections

15: Invasive procedures such as intramuscular or subcutaneous injections, suppositories or catheterisation must be avoided in the patient who is neutropenic and thrombocytopenic for the following reason:
4) All of the above

16: A skin-tunnelled catheter is used for:
4) All of the above

17: Good personal hygiene on the part of the patient is important because:
2) It reduces the risk of commensal infection

LEUKAEMIA

Palliative care
Breathlessness

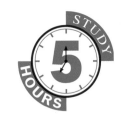

Breathlessness has been described as 'the major part of total respiratory distress, which would encompass the physical, psychological and social manifestations'.[1] Definitions, however, cannot describe the reality of breathlessness. 'It feels like you are breathing through cotton wool,' one patient has said.

Breathlessness is the presenting complaint in 10%–15% of patients with lung cancer, and occurs in up to 65% of patients at some time in their illness.[2]

An important first step in the management of breathlessness is understanding that the condition can easily become the dominant factor in a person's life, and that it may carry significant meaning for the patient.

People experiencing breathlessness as a result of lung cancer or metastatic disease frequently perceive it as a sign that they are about to die or as a reminder that death is the inevitable outcome of their illness. Managing breathlessness in patients with cancer therefore requires nurses to understand the scope of what breathlessness means to each patient. This is particularly true when breathlessness is accompanied by panic. Management of the condition involves a combination of practical measures and interpersonal approaches.

MANAGING BREATHLESSNESS

Understanding breathlessness, identifying the goals of intervention and agreeing a management strategy should always begin with dialogue with the patient. Understanding deepens over time, and extended dialogue provides the means for reflection and evaluation of an agreed care plan.

However, there are indications that breathlessness in cancer is not always well controlled by conventional means. One study assessed symptom control provided by terminal care support teams.[3] Researchers found that pain was the most common symptom at referral, but assessment scores improved after the first week of care and in the last week of life.

In contrast, all the patients with breathlessness at referral were breathless when they died, and some patients additionally developed breathlessness after referral. The researchers conclude that, despite a range of treatments including opioids, bronchodilators, anxiolytics and corticosteroids, 'dyspnoea was not controlled: existing measures may have poor efficacy or may be applied too late'.

Another study of the effectiveness of symptom control in non-small-cell lung cancer found that, despite 'appropriate conventional treatment, palliation is variable, with haemoptysis and chest pain well controlled but cough and breathlessness much less so'.[4]

Fig 1. Breathing control: using the lower abdomen

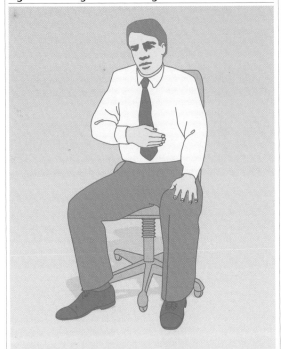

- Sit in a comfortable position with your head and back supported;

- Let your shoulders relax and fall;

- Place your hand flat on the abdomen and give a little cough. The muscle you feel under your hand is your diaphragm;

- Breathe in and gently push your abdomen or belly out (your hand will move at the same time);

- Try breathing in through your nose and out gently through your mouth as you do this, making your breath out twice as long as your breath in (counting one as you breathe in then two as you breathe out will help you);

- Remember, your belly goes out as you breathe in and in as you breathe out;

- Practise the exercise several times during the day (five to 10 breaths each time you practise is a good guideline, but adjust this as it suits you);

- In time it may be possible also to push the lower ribs out while breathing in, as well as the abdomen. This provides greater lower chest expansion than using the abdomen alone.

The causes of breathlessness in lung cancer include: asthma; chronic obstructive airway disease; collapse of the lung because of tumour obstruction of a major airway; pleural effusion (fluid between the lung and the chest wall); infection of the lung; pulmonary embolism; pericardial effusion; and lymphangitis carcinaomatosa (diffuse tumour invasion of the small lymphatics of the lung).[5]

If airway obstruction is incomplete, the patient may develop a wheeze that becomes worse in deep breathing, especially while exercising. Deep breathing in these cases may exacerbate shortness of breath and cause discomfort or pain. Gentle regular breathing is much less distressing.

Similarly, advising patients to sit with their upper body angled forward and supported during episodes of breathlessness may not be appropriate for patients with malignant disease. These patients may respond better to a more upright posture, either leaning back against a wall or seated, hands resting just above the knees with their back upright. The objective is to find a position that is comfortable for the individual.

MEDICAL APPROACHES

From a medical point of view, each of the distinct causes of breathlessness requires a distinct treatment or palliation.[1]

Radiotherapy is an important treatment for cancer-related breathlessness: an obstructed bronchus can often be re-opened after a single dose of radiotherapy. Studies have shown that a range of symptoms — cough, haemoptysis, chest pain, anorexia, and dysphagia — can be palliated in this way in most patients.[6] The use of chemotherapy in the relief of breathlessness is less widespread.

The roles of hypoxia and oxygen therapy in breathlessness from cancer are disputed. It is claimed that the majority of patients with malignant causes for breathlessness do not require oxygen therapy to correct hypoxia.[6] But it has been found that most cancer patients seem to have dyspnoea associated with hypoxia.[7] Furthermore, supplemental oxygen has been shown to reduce dyspnoea in cancer patients who are hypoxic and breathless at rest and, even when unrelated to hypoxia, symptomatic relief has been demonstrated through the use of oxygen.[7] Administering oxygen therapy almost always involves significant restrictions on a person's freedom of movement, speech and ability to eat and drink. A table fan to direct airflow across the face has also been suggested as helpful.[1]

Pleural effusion is a frequent cause of breathlessness in cancer: it is most effectively treated by pleural aspiration.[1] Following aspiration, a sclerosing agent such as bleomycin or tetracycline may be introduced into the pleural space to make the two surfaces stick together.

DRUG TREATMENTS

A number of drug treatments are commonly used for the relief of breathlessness in cancer, although it is recognised that no single treatment can be overwhelmingly helpful.

Bronchodilators may be useful for patients whose breathlessness is exacerbated by reversible airways disease: reversibility is assessed by measuring the patient's peak expiratory flow rate (PEFR) before and after a standard dose of a prescribed bronchodilator, such as salbutamol. An improvement of more than 15% suggest that the patient will derive significant benefit from the use of such drugs.[7]

Respiratory sedatives, most commonly morphine, are frequently recommended to alleviate breathlessness in advanced cancer. The effect of morphine in breathlessness is not well understood. However, opiates have been shown to increase substantially the exercise capacity of patients with chronic obstructive pulmonary disease[8] and 'most palliative care physicians now agree that low-dose systemic opioids have a place in the symptomatic management of breathlessness in patients with malignant disease.'[9]

NURSING APPROACHES

To manage the physical effects of breathlessness and to try to understand and alleviate the mental distress of breathlessness in life-threatening disease, researchers and practitioners at the Centre for Cancer and Palliative Care Studies established a nurse-led clinic for patients in a London cancer unit.[10,11]

More recently, work has been under way in conjunction with the Macmillan Practice Development Unit to introduce similar clinics in a number of hospitals in England and Wales.[12] The nurse-led clinic offers patients a package of care designed to respond to breathlessness in an integrated way.

Patients (and a partner or friend) are invited to attend the clinic for about an hour each week for an initial period of eight weeks. This gives nurses and patients the chance to review the impact of breathlessness on the patient so that intervention can be integrated with daily life.

Assessment reveals what makes breathlessness worse, and also what makes it better for the patient. Often, the way daily activities are carried out can be modified to remove unnecessary demands on respiration.

Adapting to being breathless
For instance, patients can be advised to remain sitting for as much time as possible while dressing, and to wear loose-fitting clothes, especially around the waist and chest. Bending over at the waist when putting on socks, tights and shoes could be avoided by bending at the knee. Resisting the temptation to hold one's breath when pulling off clothes may be helpful too.

Rushing to answer the telephone, or standing while on the telephone, can exacerbate breathlessness. Pausing before speaking and after each sentence can make conversations easier.

Showering and bathing may be particularly worrying

to a patient. If the weather permits, opening a window slightly can help this. Other suggestions include bathing in quite shallow and not very hot water.

The process of getting in and out of the bath can be reconfigured: having undressed, patients can be advised to sit at the side of the bath and slowly lift one leg in at a time; when getting out, it may be easier first to move into a kneeling position.

Having sex may be easier if patients and their partners become more aware of exactly what activities result in shortness of breath. Positions that minimise breathlessness can be suggested. For example, it may be easier to adopt a sitting position. It may be difficult for someone who is breathless to lie underneath his or her partner: a standing position may be easier.

Detailed consideration of breathlessness with patients, including the feelings it evokes and the changes it brings, provides an opportunity to both understand it and prepare for it.

One means of preparing for breathlessness is breathing retraining. The aims of breathing retraining, which was originally developed for patients with chronic respiratory disease, are shown in the box above.

BREATHING RETRAINING

Breathing retraining consists of a number of separate techniques, including diaphragmatic breathing (or breathing control, Fig 1).[13] Often breathlessness can lead a person to breathe with the upper chest and shoulders in a rapid, shallow manner. Gasping for air increases the resistance to flow, which increases energy expenditure. Using accessory muscles, which are not as efficient as primary respiratory muscles, quickly leads to fatigue and to greater oxygen consumption. As the rate of breathing increases, the depth often decreases, creating a larger dead space in the lungs and reducing the amount of oxygen available to the body. In effect, this response to inadequate ventilation actually places even greater demands on the respiratory system.[14]

Breathing control, in which the patient uses the diaphragm, the abdominal muscles, scalenes and intercostal muscles, is used at rest or to avoid breathlessness or exertion (Fig 1).[13]

Over a course of weekly sessions, patient and nurse can work on improving this technique and move on to using it while walking, climbing stairs (breathing in climbing one step and out and climbing the next) and performing agreed activities.

Given the trust and permission of the patient, the nurse may be able to demonstrate, by gently touching the patient's shoulders, how rapid shallow breaths and tense, bunched shoulders have become the established pattern of respiration. Often this contact is in itself soothing. It will also provide a breathing pattern baseline to be compared with the more controlled patterns of respiration that emerge as breathing retraining continues (see Box 1).

Using the diaphragm and lower chest muscles to assist respiration provides some with means of managing the panic associated with acute episodes of increased shortness of breath as well as a strategy gradually to expand the patient's circle of activities.

A type of breathing economy may develop in which realistic, priority activities are contemplated. Planning activities to avoid unnecessary expenditure of energy, and pacing them — attempting only as many as can be comfortably achieved each day — focuses patients on the activities that mean most to them.

MANAGING PANIC

Managing the panic associated with breathlessness almost always requires dialogue to explore the fears that lead to the panic, and that in turn often leads the patient to acknowledging the fear of cancer itself.

The reality of breathlessness in lung cancer may force the patient both into a radical reformulation of what it is possible to do on a day-to-day basis and bring to the fore fears relating to suffocation and life-threatening disease.

Supporting patients experiencing breathlessness in this way involves providing a forum for fears to be expressed: breathlessness is alleviated by allowing the fear it causes to be talked about.

Psychotherapeutically speaking, this means 'being there for the patient', or 'allowing the patient, to some extent, to use the nurse symbolically as a container for whatever of his or her anxieties are, at the moment, intolerable to him or her'.[15]

Working in this way, however, is stressful for nurses. It can be successfully undertaken only under the guidance of practitioners with the relevant expertise and within a system of clinical supervision or reflective practice with a facilitator. In this way the feelings aroused in close relationships with distressed patients can themselves be supported and contained.

A study to evaluate the effectiveness of the package of care offered in the nurse-led clinic provided encouraging signs that the management of breathlessness in lung cancer could be improved considerably. Median scores for breathlessness at worst, distress due to breathlessness, functional capacity and difficulty in performing activities of daily living all improved for patients receiving the intervention.

Strategies focused on both functional and personal aspects of the condition provide the opportunity to take the management of breathlessness in cancer forward.

The evidence provided by the nurse-led clinic means that there is now scope for cautious optimism that breathlessness in lung cancer is not beyond the scope of nursing intervention. Combining dialogue and partnership with skilled application of techniques of breathing retraining has led to a management strategy with the potential to provide tangible improvements in quality of life.

Partnership and dialogue with other units caring for patients with similar needs holds out the prospect of more widespread innovation in practice. If we refuse to accept that the boundaries of established care and treatment are the boundaries of all possible care and treatment, nursing practice will have the room to develop and grow, especially in those areas where nursing care has sometimes been thought to have little to offer.

THINKING POINTS

● Can you remember a time when you felt that you could not breathe? How would you describe the feeling?
● What issues do the above findings raise about existing approaches to symptom management in advanced cancer?

PART TWO

Nausea and vomiting

Patients with advanced illnesses frequently experience nausea and vomiting. These symptoms can be demoralising and demeaning,[16] and failure to relieve them diminishes patients' quality of life and may exacerbate the pain and distress of friends and relatives.[17] The successful management of these symptoms is therefore clearly of the utmost importance.

Nausea has been described as an unpleasant sensation, located in the gastrointestinal region, which may also be accompanied by the urge to vomit.[18] It can also be a total body sensation. Vomiting is the forceful expulsion of gastro-intestinal contents (Fig 2).

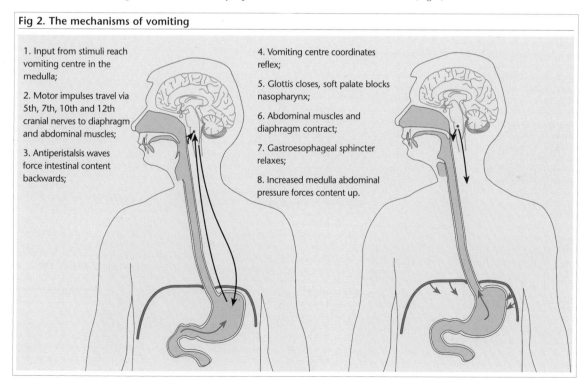

Fig 2. The mechanisms of vomiting

1. Input from stimuli reach vomiting centre in the medulla;

2. Motor impulses travel via 5th, 7th, 10th and 12th cranial nerves to diaphragm and abdominal muscles;

3. Antiperistalsis waves force intestinal content backwards;

4. Vomiting centre coordinates reflex;

5. Glottis closes, soft palate blocks nasopharynx;

6. Abdominal muscles and diaphragm contract;

7. Gastroesophageal sphincter relaxes;

8. Increased medulla abdominal pressure forces content up.

PALLIATIVE CARE

Table 1. Assessment of the causes of nausea and vomiting

Assessment	Gastro-intestinal stasis	Positional/movement	Cerebral	Chemical	Emotional
Frequency	Infrequent	On movement	Variable	Often	Related to trigger
Volume	Large	Small	Small	Small	Small
Nausea	✔	✔	✔	✔	✔
Timing	May vary	Related to movement	May be worse in the morning	Variable trigger factors	Related to emotions
Nature/ associated factors	Vomit is composed of foul food	N/a	Sleepy/headache Neurological signs Headaches and vomiting	Associated symptoms of: Hypercalcaemia Uraemia Newly-commenced drugs Radiotherapy Chemotherapy	Phobias Anxiety Fear Anticipatory nausea and vomiting Memories

Table 2. Causes of nausea and vomiting in advanced illness

Drug/treatment-induced vomiting	Opioids; iron supplements; antibiotics; cytotoxic agents; corticosteroids; non-steroidal anti-inflammatory drugs; radiotherapy especially when the field of treatment includes the brain or the gastro-intestinal tract
Disease-related causes	Gastric irritation; constipation; electrolyte/metabolic disturbances such as uraemia and hypercalcaemia, hyponatraemia and ketosis; raised intracranial pressures; gastro-intestinal obstruction; hepatomegaly; squashed stomach syndrome
Psychological causes	Anxiety; fear; phobias (for example, fear of hypodermic needles); sights; odours

One author suggests that 30% of people with terminal illness experience vomiting and 60% experience nausea.[16] A recent small-scale study examining the side-effects of the chemotherapeutic agent carboplatin found that the mean incidence of nausea in this group was 69% and the mean incidence of vomiting was 25%.[19] In a survey of 200 consecutive admissions to a palliative care unit, it was found that 30% of patients experienced nausea and vomiting.[20] It has also been suggested that patients who experience nausea and dyspnoea suffer more pain than patients who do not.[21]

Much research has been directed towards the successful management of nausea and vomiting associated with chemotherapy. Such attention is justifiable but more attention now needs to be paid to nausea and vomiting in advanced illness, where multiple causes often pose a unique challenge to symptom relief.

ASSESSMENT

Advanced illness brings with it a number of disease or treatment-related factors which may combine to produce nausea and vomiting to varying degrees.[22] The decision surrounding the choice of antiemetic is complex and is influenced by a variety of causative factors.[23]

The interrelated causes demand meticulous assessment, the aim of which is to ensure the right intervention is given at the right time for a clearly defined reason. Nurses providing palliative care are in an ideal position to offer much of the information needed for an accurate appraisal of the cause or causes.

TOOLS FOR ASSESSMENT

As with the monitoring of pain, nausea can be assessed using visual analogue scales. However, the factors that cause nausea and vomiting in advanced illness change as the illness progresses, and the patient's capacity to use these scales decreases. Communication difficulties, fatigue and confusion may pose problems in the use of the scales as an accurate measure of the intensity of the patient's nausea.[24]

Patterns of nausea and vomiting may be significant in helping to pinpoint the cause (Table 1). The general causes of nausea and vomiting in advanced illness are outlined in Table 2. Although full investigation of the causes of nausea and vomiting is essentially the remit of the medical team, nurses have a role in symptom assessment and in the planning, implementation and evaluation of care. This role is becoming more prominent in the light of developing specialist nursing posts in palliative care.

PHARMACOLOGICAL MANAGEMENT

The vomiting centre is situated in the reticular formation of the brain. The emetic response is instigated when it receives stimuli from the abdominal organs, the cerebral cortex, the chemoreceptor trigger and the vestibular centres (Fig 3).[25]

When examining the causes of nausea and vomiting it becomes obvious that a wide range of causes relate to altered biochemical and mechanical functions. This implies that pharmacological intervention may be appropriate for a majority of patients.

Twycross and Lack[18] suggest that antiemetics should be prescribed according to the following criteria:
● The cause of nausea and vomiting;
● The affinity of the drug with the neurotransmitter sites;
● The preferred route of administration.

It is estimated that up to 25% of patients will need two antiemetics to control nausea and vomiting.[26] Regnard suggests a single antiemetic is sufficient in two-thirds of patients.[27]

When secondary drugs have to be offered, it is important that they have a different mode of action.[16, 27] However, occasionally, combinations of drugs with a similar action, such as metoclopramide with domperidone, can be effective.

A systematic and incremental approach to tackling persistent problems is important. A suggested framework is carefully to assess the severity of the problem and, where possible, identify the most likely cause.[28]

Where identified, potentially reversible causes such as constipation, hypercalcaemia or severe pain should be treated first before giving antiemetic agents. Give an appropriate first-line antiemetic regularly and offer extra doses if necessary.

If the patient is vomiting more than three times in 24 hours or within two hours of taking oral medication or is nauseated most of the time, the drug can be given parenterally or by continuous subcutaneous infusion. The dose can be adjusted every 24 hours as necessary. If there is little or no improvement after 24 to 48 hours, reassessment is needed to ensure that the right cause is being addressed. If it is not, a different antiemetic should be used. If the right cause is not being addressed, further assessment is necessary. Hawthorn[29] mentions that steroids have been shown to enhance the role of metoclopramide.

If reasonable control is achieved after 72 hours of parenteral medication, an equivalent oral regime can be considered.

Advanced illness may mean the patient cannot take

Table 3. Medications used in the management of nausea and vomiting and in advanced illness

Metoclopran	This has a weak central action but because it increases gastric mobility it is useful in dealing with gastro-intestinal causes of nausea and vomiting, such as gastric stasis;
Ondansetron	This may be the first drug of choice in the management of nausea and vomiting induced by chemotherapy.[30] It is a specific antagonist of SHT receptors associated with the central connections of the vagus nerve in the brainstem in close proximity to the chemoreceptor trigger zone;
Corticosteroids	These are of value in the management of nausea and vomiting related to enlarged organs though their anti-inflammatory effect. Dexamethane is particularly useful in managing nausea and vomiting resulting from tumour-induced cerebral oedema;
Domperidone	This acts on the gut wall and may be of value in dealing with oesophageal reflux. The drug had been identified as being ineffective in opioid-induced vomiting;[31]
Octreotide	This is a recent addition. It is used principally in the management of nausea and vomiting associated with bowel obstruction in terminal disease. Riley and Fallon observed a reduction in vomiting and pain as well as improvement in a sense of well-being following the use of the drug.[16] It is usually given by subcutaneous injection;
Haloperidol	This is a dopamine receptor antagonist that reduces the sensitivity of the chemoreceptor trigger zone to a range of biochemical stimuli, for example opioids and uraemia;
Cyclizine	This is an antihistamine that is of value in advanced vomiting.[5] This drug may also be indicated where vestibular disturbances or radiotherapy to the head and neck may be the source of nausea and vomiting. Williams suggests it may be of value in managing emesis from intestinal obstruction;[22]
Hyoscine	This is an anticholinergic, an agent that inhibits nerve impulse transmission. It is thought to act as a depressant on the vomiting centre.[29] It dries the secretions so may reduce retching in a patients who has excessive bronchial secretions.

Fig 1. Pathways that instigate the emetic response

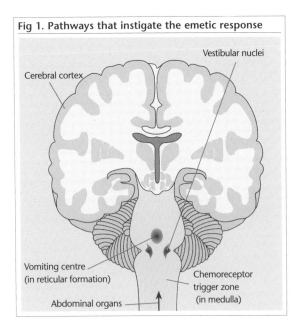

Labels: Vestibular nuclei; Cerebral cortex; Vomiting centre (in reticular formation); Abdominal organs; Chemoreceptor trigger zone (in medulla)

oral medication but intravenous antiemetic therapy may not be appropriate. In this case, the drugs can be given via suppository or syringe driver.

Prochlorperazine, cyclizine, domperidone and chlorpromazine are examples of drugs that may be given in suppository form.

In severe vomiting where oral medication is inappropriate, cyclizine, metoclopramide, octreotide and haloperidol can be administered subcutaneously.

The increasing range of modes for delivering antiemetics has been of particular value to practitioners involved in palliative care in the community. The drugs commonly used in the management of nausea and vomiting are outlined in Table 3.

NON-PHARMACOLOGICAL APPROACHES

The successful management of nausea and vomiting remains a challenge for practitioners engaged in palliative care. There are a number of moral issues that make it difficult to establish comparative trials of antiemetic regimes in patients with advanced illness. These should not prevent the systematic review of the effectiveness of approaches in managing nausea and vomiting. More work needs to be done on developing tools for assessing nausea and vomiting that are sensitive to the unique problems faced by patients with advanced illness.

The emergence of treatments such as hypnosis, progressive muscle relaxation and imagery techniques have enlarged the repertoire of interventions that can be used in conjunction with drugs to deal with nausea and vomiting.[30]

While neither pharmacology nor complementary approaches alone hold the key to successful management of these symptoms, used together, control of emesis may become a more realistic goal.

A majority of complementary therapies interfere with conditioning stimuli, such as sights, sounds and smells, which may initiate or sustain the emetic response. Anxiety associated with advanced illness may itself cause nausea or exacerbate its intensity. Complementary therapies may reduce anxiety, therefore reducing the psychological component of nausea and vomiting.

Nursing and medical audit and the sharing of data are likely to provide more information to ensure our effectiveness in managing these difficult symptoms. The potential development of specialist and advanced practitioners in palliative care will require that nurses have an in-depth knowledge of the theory and practice of emesis management.

THINKING POINTS

● What kind of assessment scheme do you use to assess nausea and vomiting in terminally ill patients? What makes assessing the causes of nausea and vomiting in terminal illness so difficult?
● Which non-pharmacological approaches could be used as effective adjuvants to drug therapy in managing nausea and vomiting? What are the advantages and disadvantages of using non-pharmacological approaches?

PART THREE

Pain

Pain is neither the most common problem in those with cancer nor the most difficult to manage, yet it is the most feared symptom.

It is perceived by nurses to be the most distressing symptom in people with cancer[33] and, often, the greatest fear of the dying and their families is pain. However, cancer pain can be managed successfully.

Pain is a somatopsychic experience: 'An unpleasant sensory and emotional experience associated with actual or potential tissue damage, or described in terms of such damage'.[34] It is a complex phenomenon, with many factors contributing to a person's perception of it. Both psychological and physical factors interact to produce the 'total pain' experience. This concept of total pain was first used by Saunders[35] in reference to physical, social, emotional and spiritual pain, and since then has been recognised as important in helping to understand the complexity of the feelings experienced by cancer patients.

INCIDENCE

Although the exact incidence of cancer pain is currently unknown, studies looking at its incidence and severity suggest that between 55% to 95% of patients with advanced cancer experience pain, with 20% to 50% of patients experiencing pain at diagnosis.[36]

The amount of pain that a person with cancer experiences varies according to the primary site of their cancer. Hanks' study found that fewer patients with leukaemia (<10%) are likely to have severe pain than those with bone or cervical cancer (>80%).[37]

However, pain and cancer are not synonymous. Approximately 75% of patients with advanced cancer experience pain, the rest do not. About a third of patients feeling pain will have only one pain, the rest will have two or more concurrent pains.[38]

THE NATURE OF PAIN

The physical pain experienced by patients with cancer can be divided into four categories:
● Caused by the cancer itself;
● Related to treatment;
● Related to cancer and/or debility;
● Incidental/benign causes.[39]

The most common cause of pain in cancer is that from the cancer itself, mainly bone, visceral, neuropathic and soft tissue pain.[38] Not all pain experienced is due to the cancer. Twycross and Lack suggest that 33% of pain experienced by cancer patients is incidental, for example from arthritis.[40] Pain can also be related to treatment; for instance, from constipation due to analgesic therapy or as a result of treatment itself, for example, post-radiotherapy fibrosis.

Emotional and social pain
Pain is rarely caused entirely by non-physical means, but emotional and social problems often intensify a patient's experience of pain. A person's past experience of pain may affect his/her current perception of it.[41]

People who have previously had pain that has been uncontrolled may feel apprehensive and fearful. Those with increased distress, for example fear, frustration and anger, report more pain. These are common emotions in people coming to terms with cancer but they may also have a fear of hospitals, pain and death, or of what will happen to their family and friends.[40]

Good communication between nurses and patients, and between patients and families, is essential as lack of communication can cause misunderstanding and fear, thus increasing distress and having an adverse effect on their experience of pain.

Culture and upbringing may affect the way people perceive their pain. If they are raised in a culture that accepts and encourages the outward expression of pain, they will be expressive in describing their pain and this can lower their pain threshold.

Although anecdotal evidence suggests that there may be a gender difference in how people respond to pain, there is no consensus in the literature either way.

SPIRITUAL PAIN

Most dying patients will be affected by spiritual pain at some stage of their illness. Few people will show doubts and grief in distinct religious ways, but feelings of guilt and worthlessness are forms of spiritual pain.

The meaning of pain is important to a person's perception of it. If the pain serves some purpose and is a consequence of a disease process that can be cured, the person is more likely to cope with it than is someone whose pain is a constant reminder of a disease that will lead to that person's death.

The pain of dying patients causes distress both to them and to their family and is a constant reminder that they have cancer and are going to die.[38] Clearly, then, a priority in the nursing care of the terminally ill is to manage their pain thus improving their quality of life.

PAIN ASSESSMENT

The assessment of pain is important for effective control and is an essential part of nursing care. Nurses are ideally placed to do this and to evaluate the success of any analgesics or interventions given. They need to be aware of ways of measuring pain and the importance of documenting this; Camp and O'Sullivan found that nurses documented significantly less than 50% of the pain that patients described.[10]

Most departments use a pain assessment tool to help in assessment and documentation. Assessment tools come in a variety of forms, including pain scales, body diagrams and questionnaires.

Since patients with cancer rarely have only one site of pain, it is important that each site is assessed separately, as one site may respond to treatment while another does not.

Assessment tools must be used over a period of time in order to build up a picture of the pain and also to evaluate interventions given. Ideally, pain assessment forms should be filled in by patients, as only they can accurately describe the pain. This may not always be possible, though, for if they are in severe pain they may be in no state to fill in forms.

The most common assessment tools contain a mixture of scales, body diagrams and questions in order to get as complete a picture as possible. They may include a visual analogue scale. In their simplest form such scales

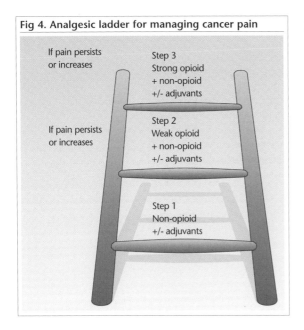

Fig 4. Analgesic ladder for managing cancer pain

If pain persists or increases

Step 3
Strong opioid
+ non-opioid
+/- adjuvants

If pain persists or increases

Step 2
Weak opioid
+ non-opioid
+/- adjuvants

Step 1
Non-opioid
+/- adjuvants

have a horizontal or vertical line with 'no pain' written at one end and 'worst possible pain' at the other, and patients are asked to put a mark on the line between these two criteria at a position that describes their pain. Some scales will have numbers one to 10, on them, to help patients make their assessment. The marks down the scales can then be compared with future assessments to see if the pain has improved or not.

Body diagrams are useful in ascertaining where patients are experiencing pain. They are given a diagram of the front and back views of the body and are asked to mark in the areas where they are experiencing pain. This illustration can then be used to identify new areas of pain.

It is also important to get answers to questions such as, what makes your pain worse or better? Are you pain-free at rest? What analgesics are you taking?

PAIN MANAGEMENT

Management should include a diagnosis of the cause of the pain, and treatment should be individualised and specific for each patient and kept simple.

The aim of management is progressive, involving three stages. First ensuring that the patient is pain-free at night, then during the day while resting and finally on movement.[38]

Management can be split into two main areas, used simultaneously: pharmacological and non-pharmacological.

PHARMACOLOGICAL PAIN MANAGEMENT

Drugs are the most obvious form of pain control. It is important that the right drug is given at the correct dose and on the appropriate time scale.[38]

Analgesia is best given orally if possible and should be given regularly and prophylactically,[38, 43] with the interval based on the duration of analgesic effect so that the pain does not return.

The WHO suggests an analgesic ladder for the management of cancer pain (Fig 4).[43] If a drug at a given level fails to relieve the pain, then treatment moves on to the next level. Thus individual treatment is given to each patient with progressively more potent drugs until the pain is controlled.

Three groups of analgesic drugs are used, non-opioids, weak opioids and strong opioids. These are supplemented with adjuvant drugs.

Non-opioids

The main non-opioids used are paracetamol and non-steroidal anti-inflammatory drugs (NSAIDs). They are step 1 analgesics and have a 'ceiling' effect in that once the maximum effective dose has been reached, increasing the dose will not increase the analgesia. If a patient's pain is not adequately controlled, the drugs must be changed or supplemented with adjuvant drugs or opioids. Because of their inflammatory effect, NSAIDs are very useful for bone and soft tissue pains, and are used alongside the opioids.

Weak opioids

Codeine, dihydrocodeine and tramadol are all weak opioids. Codeine is less potent than morphine, and is well absorbed, but often causes constipation. Dihydrocodeine is similarly potent but causes a higher incidence of adverse effects. Tramadol is a relatively new drug and is given by mouth or injection. It is twice as strong as codeine[38] and is thought to produce less constipation and respiratory depression than conventional opioids.

Strong opioids

The most well known and widely used opiate is morphine. Oral morphine is the strong opioid of choice for cancer pain and can be administered as immediate-release tablets (for example Sevredol), in aqueous solution (such as Oramorph) and in sustained-release preparations (for instance, MXL, a once-a-day morphine preparation or MST, a twice-a-day preparation).

Immediate-release preparations should be given four-hourly and patients are encouraged to take additional rescue doses if the pain is not adequately relieved or if it returns before the next dose is due. A double dose of immediate-release morphine can be taken at bedtime.[38]

The dose of morphine should be titrated upwards using immediate release preparations until pain relief is achieved. Only then should patients be given sustained release preparations.

Opioids have several undesirable side-effects:
● Constipation, which can be more difficult to treat than the pain itself;
● Nausea and vomiting (see 'Nausea and vomiting'); regular antiemetics should be given if this develops;

● Respiratory depression; but as pain is a physiological antagonist of morphine's depressive effect, as long as the patient has pain, the dose can be safely increased without any fear of respiratory depression.[38]

Opioids are flexible in that they can be given by a variety of routes: orally, sublingually, rectally, intravenously, intramuscularly, subcutaneously and transdermally. Diamorphine hydrochloride is more soluble than morphine and is used when injections are necessary, as large amounts can be given in small volumes.

Syringe drivers are often used to give analgesia continuously via the subcutaneous route, avoiding the problem of repeated injections. When converting a patient to using a syringe driver, nurses must remember to give a 'loading' dose to cover the patient for the initial period while plasma concentrations are being built up.

A recent development in pain management has been the introduction of transdermal patches containing fentanyl. This is an opioid 80–100 times more potent than morphine and less likely to cause nausea and vomiting. The patch is designed to release fentanyl continuously and systemically for 72 hours. The patches do not allow for rapid dose titration owing to the slow onset of action, and immediate-release morphine may be needed for analgesic cover during the first 6–12 hours, until the plasma concentration has built up.

If a patient is to be changed from one opioid to another, the dose of drug must be converted to an equianalgesic dose. For example, if a patient is on buprenorphine 1.2mg daily, the conversion factor is x50, so they are on the equivalent of 60mg oral morphine daily.

Likewise, changing the route of administration, for example intravenous to oral, the parenteral:oral ratio must be taken into account in order to calculate the conversion from an intravenous to an oral dose. Conversion tables are available for calculating equianalgesic doses.

Adjuvant medication
Adjuvant therapy is an important part of pain management. An adjuvant drug is one that potentiates the activity of another. These drugs can help to allay pains unresponsive to opioids or to support procedures such as radiotherapy. Examples of adjuvant drugs are tricyclic antidepressants, neuroleptics, muscle relaxants and steroids.

NON-PHARMACOLOGICAL MANAGEMENT

Non-pharmacological pain management can be divided into primary methods, which eliminate or reduce the cause of pain and secondary methods, which eliminate or reduce pain, or increase pain tolerance.

Primary methods
Neurological and neurosurgical interventions involve an interruption of pain pathways. Generally, nerve blocks are best suited to patients with a short life-expectancy and

these who have well-localised pain that has proved difficult to control.

Radiotherapy modifies the pathological process of cancer, while external beam radiotherapy is a standard treatment for painful bone metastases.

Secondary methods
Relaxation aims to reduce anxiety and tension and to promote an increased sense of control so that patients can cope better with their pain.[33] Distraction will focus a patient's attention away from the pain and here techniques such as music therapy have been used successfully.[44]

There are numerous reports of the successful use of hypnosis in cancer pain, but much of the evidence is inadequate.[33]

Physical methods of pain relief include support and positioning, superficial heat and cold application, massage and touch and transcutaneous electrical nerve stimulation (TENS).[33] Good communication is vital when caring for the terminally ill. Time spent talking to a patient can increase the person's pain threshold. If psychological factors are ignored, pain may become intractable.

Other methods of non-pharmacological pain control include acupuncture, imagery, breathing techniques and Yoga.

All these methods of non-pharmacological pain control can be used in conjunction with each other but they are complementary to analgesics and do not replace them.

CONCLUSION

Nurses need to be able to establish a rapport with patients so that they can tackle the problem of pain together. They need to be familiar with the use of assessment tools and with the different factors that affect patients' total experience of their pain.

An understanding of the different methods of pain control is also important so that treatment and strategies can be explained to patients and their families. Nurses thus can act as advocates in ensuring that their patients get the best possible pain management.

Management of pain in terminally ill cancer patients is possible: a third of patients with advanced cancer do not experience pain and of the remaining two-thirds, pain relief can be achieved in nine out of 10 of such patients.[33]

THINKING POINT

● How would you describe the different kinds of pain described to you by patients you have cared for? What were the different causes for the pain they described?
● What strategies do you employ for assessing pain? How effective do you think they are?

REFERENCES

1. Doyle D., Hanks, G.W.C., MacDonald, N. *Oxford Textbook of Palliative Medicine*. Oxford: Oxford University Press, 1993.
2. Reuben, B.B., Mor, V. Dyspnoea in terminally ill cancer patients. *Chest* 1986; 89: 2, 234-236.
3. Higginson, I., McCarthy, M. Measuring symptoms in terminal cancer: are pain and dyspnoea controlled? *Journal of the Royal Society of Medicine* 1989; 82: 264-267.
4. Muers, M.F., Round,C.E. Palliation of symptoms in non-small cell lung cancer: a study by the Yorkshire Regional Cancer Organisation thoracic group. *Thorax* 1993; 48: 339-343.
5. Cowcher, K., Hanks,G.W. Long-term management of respiratory symptoms in advanced cancer. *Journal of Pain and Symptom Management* 1990; 5: 5, 320-330.
6. Ahmedzai, S. Respiratory distress in the terminally ill. *Respiratory Disease in Practice* 1988; October/November, 20-29.
7. Walsh, D. Dyspnoea in advanced cancer. *The Lancet* 1993; 342: 450-451.
8 Light, R.W., Muro, J.R., Sato, R.I., et al. Effects of oral morphine on breathlessness. *American Review of Respiratory Diseases* 1989; 139: 126-133.
9. Davis, C.L. The therapeutics of dyspnoea. In: *Cancer Surveys Volume 21: Palliative Medicine Problem Areas in Pain and Symptom Management*. London: Imperial Cancer Research Fund, 1994.
10. Corner, J., Plant, H., Warner, L. Developing a nursing approach to managing dyspnoea in lung cancer. *International Journal of Palliative Nursing* 1995; **1**: 1.
11. Corner, J., Plant, H., A'Hern, R., Bailey, C. Non-pharmacological intervention for breathlessness in lung cancer. *Palliative Medicine* 1996; 10: 4, 299-306.
12. Bailey, C. Ethical issues in multicentre collaborative research on breathlessness in lung cancer. *International Journal of Palliative Nursing* 1996; 2: 2, 95-101.
13. Webber, B. The role of the physiotherapist in medical chest problems. *Respiratory Disease in Practice* 1991; February/March, 12-15.
14. Gift, A.G., Cahill, C.A. Psychophysiologic aspects of dyspnoea in chronic obstructive pulmonary disease: a pilot study. *Heart and Lung* 1990; 19: 3, 252-257.
15. Fabricius, J. Running on the spot or can nursing really change? *Psychoanalytic Psychotherapy* 1991; 5: 2, 97-108.
16. Allan, S.G. Nausea and vomiting. In: Doyle, D, Hanks, G.W.C., McDonald, N. (eds). *Oxford Textbook of Palliative Medicine*. Oxford: Oxford University Press, 1993.
17. Outwerkerk, J., Keizer, H. Psychological aspects of the treatment of cancer. *Seminars in Oncology Nursing* 1990; 6: 4, Suppl 1, 6-7.
18. Twycross, R., Lack. S. *Therapeutics in Terminal Cancer*. Edinburgh: Churchill Livingstone, 1990.
19. Buckingham, R., Fitt, J., Sitzia, J. Patients' experience of chemotherapy. *European Journal of Cancer Care* 1997; 6: 1, 59-71.
20. Finlay, I. The management of other frequently encountered symptoms. In: Penson J., Fisher, R. (eds). *Palliative Care for People with Cancer*. London: Edward Arnold, 1991.
21. Desbiens, N.A., Rizner-Mueller, N., Connors, A.F., et al. The relationship of nausea and dyspnoea to pain in seriously ill patients. *Pain* 1997; 71: 2, 49-156.
22. Regnard, C., Comiskey, M. Nausea and vomiting in advanced cancer. *Palliative Medicine* 1992; **6**: 2, 146-151.
23. Redmond, K. Advances in supportive care. *European Journal of Cancer Care* 1996; 5: suppl 2, 1-7.
24. Borjescu et al. Similarities and differences in assessing nausea in a verbal category scale and a visual analogue scale. *Cancer Nursing* 1997; 20: 4, 260-266.
25. Pilsworth, T., Pye, D., Roberts, A. Symptom control in advanced cancer. In: Dvud, J. (ed). *Cancer Care Prevention. Treatment and palliation*. London: Chapman & Hall, 1995.
26. Kay, P. *A-Z Pocket Book of Symptom Control*. Northampton: EPL Publications, 1994.
27. Regnard, C.F.B., Tempest, S. *A Guide to Symptom Relief in Advanced Cancer*. Manchester: Haigh and Hochland, 1992.
28. Twycross, R. *Introducing Palliative Care*. Oxford: Radcliffe Medical, 1997.
29. Hawthorn, J. *Understanding and Management of Nausea and Vomiting*. Oxford: Blackwell, 1995.
30. Black, P.M., Morrow, G.R. Anticipatory nausea and emesis: behavioural interventions. In: Watson, M. *Cancer Patient Care: Psychosocial treatment methods*. Cambridge: Cambridge University Press, 1991.
31. Riley, J., Fallon, M.T. Octreotide in terminal malignant obstruction of the gastrointestinal tract. *European Journal of Palliative Care* 1994; 1: 1, 23-25.
32. Williams, C. Causes and management of nausea and vomiting. *Nursing Times* 1994; 90: 44, 38-41.
33. Jandelli, K. A comparative study of patient's perceptions of pain relief. International Journal of Palliative Nursing 1995; 1: 2, 74-80.
34. International Association for the Study of Pain Task Force on Taxonomy. *Classification of Chronic Pain*. Seattle: IASP Press, 1994.
35. Saunders, C.M., Baines, M.J. *Living with Dying. The management of terminal disease*. Oxford: Oxford University Press, 1989.
36. Brescia, F. J. Pain management issues as part of the comprehensive care of the cancer patient. *Seminars in Oncology* 1993; 20: 1; suppl A, 48-52.
37. Hanks, G. Pain control in cancer patients. *Cancer Topics* 1985; 5: 5, 54-56.
38. Twycross, R. *Introducing Palliative Care*. Oxford: Radcliffe Medical Press, 1997.
39. Twycross, R. *Pain Relief in Advanced Cancer*. Edinburgh, Churchill Livingstone, 1994.
40. Twycross, R.G., Lack, S. *Therapeutics in Terminal Cancer*. New York: Churchill Livingstone, 1990.
41. Skevington, S. *Psychology of Pain*. Chichester: John Wiley and Sons, 1994.
42. Camp, L.D., O'Sullivan, P.S. Comparison of medical, surgical and oncology patients' description of pain and nurses' documentation of pain assessments. *Journal of Advanced Nursing* 1987; 12: 5, 593-598.
43. World Health Organization. *Cancer Pain Relief and Palliative Care*. Geneva: WHO, 1990.
44. Magil-Levreault, L. Music therapy: variations on a theme — music therapy in pain and symptom management. *Journal of Palliative Care* 1993; 9: 4, 42-48.

Palliative care

Assessment

When you have read the unit and completed any further reading, you can use the questions below to test your understanding of the topic. Answers can be found on the next page

1 **Breathlessness is the presenting complaint in what proportion of patients with lung cancer?**

- 1 5–10%
- 2 10–15%
- 3 45–50%
- 4 85–90%

2 **A study of symptom control in terminal care found?**

- 1 Breathlessness was the most common symptom of referral
- 2 A minority of patients were breathless when they died
- 3 Pain was less well controlled than breathlessness
- 4 Breathlessness was not controlled at all

3 **Breathlessness can cause a person to breath with:**

- 1 The diaphragm
- 2 The abdominal muscles
- 3 Reduced oxygen consumption
- 4 The upper chest and shoulders

4 **Breathing control may help to avoid breathlessness. A key part of breathing control is:**

- 1 Breathe in gently and tense the abdominal muscles
- 2 Breath in and gently push the abdomen out
- 3 Breathe in deeply and push the abdomen out
- 4 Increase the rate and depth of respiration

5 **Breathing control is used:**

- 1 Only when the patient is seated
- 2 After drug treatment had been shown to be ineffective
- 3 At the patient's discretion and in conjunction with medical treatments
- 4 Only in patients with chronic obstructive pulmonary disease

6 **The estimated percentage of terminally ill patients who experience nausea is:**

- 1 20%
- 2 30%
- 3 50%
- 4 60%

7 **The vomiting centre is located in the:**

- 1 Gastric mucosa
- 2 Cerebral cortex
- 3 Chemoreceptor trigger zone
- 4 Reticular formation of the brain

8 **Corticosteroids are useful in the management of nausea and vomiting in which of the following situations:**

- 1 Opioid-induced
- 2 Organomegaly
- 3 Gastric obstruction
- 4 The presence of cerebral metastases

9 **Which of the following profiles may indicate chemically-induced vomiting?**

- 1 Large volume, infrequent vomiting
- 2 Frequent vomiting, small volume
- 3 Small volume of vomit; may be worse in the morning
- 4 Small volume of vomit related to movement

10 **Which of the following drugs is particularly useful in managing opioid-induced vomiting?**

- 1 Haloperidol
- 2 Metoclopramide
- 3 Domperidone
- 4 Corticosteroids

11 **What percentage of patients are estimated to need at least two antiemetic drugs to control nausea and vomiting?**

- 1 10%
- 2 60%
- 3 25%
- 4 40%

PALLIATIVE CARE

12 **A patient had been taking 40mg of Sevredol 4-hourly to control pain. On changing medication to MST the dose will be converted to:**

1	40mg twice a day
2	40mg four times a day
3	120mg twice a day
4	240mg twice a day

13 **The cancer pain of a terminally ill patient is:**

1	Always related to the disease
2	Often caused by non-physical means
3	Serves a useful purpose
4	Is not always due to the cancer itself

14 **Pain assessment is:**

1	Undertaken only on admission
2	An essential part of nursing care

3	Always documented by nurses
4	Well documented by nurses

15 **Adjuvant drugs are:**

1	Used instead of analgesics
2	Drugs that always control the pain directly
3	Used in isolation
4	Used alongside analgesics

16 **Non-pharmacological methods of pain control are:**

1	Complementary to analgesics
2	Used in isolation
3	All aimed at eliminating or reducing the cause of pain
4	Use to modify the pathological process of cancer

ANSWERS

Palliative care

1: Breathlessness is the presenting complaint in what proportion of patients with lung cancer?
2) 10–15%

2: A study of symptom control in terminal care found:
4) Breathlessness was not controlled at all

3: Breathlessness can cause a person to breathe with:
4) The upper chest and shoulders

4: Breathing control may help to avoid breathlessness. A key part of breathing control is:
2) Breathe in and gently push the abdomen out

5: Breathing control is used:
3) At the patient's discretion and in conjunction with medical treatments

6: The estimated percentage of terminally ill patients who experience nausea is:
4) 60%

7: The vomiting centre is located in the:
4) Reticular formation of the brain

8: Corticosteroids are useful in the management of nausea and vomiting in which of the following situations:
2) Organomegaly

9: Which of the following profiles may indicate chemically-induced vomiting?
2) Frequent vomiting, small volume

10: Which of the following drugs is particularly useful in managing opioid-induced vomiting?
1) Haloperidol

11: What percentage of patients are estimated to need at least two antiemetic drugs to control nausea and vomiting:
3) 25%

12: A patient who has been taking 40mg of Sevredol 4-hourly to control pain. On changing medication to MST the dose will be converted to:
3) 120mg twice a day

13: The cancer pain of a terminally ill patient is:
4) Not always due to the cancer itself

14: The pain assessment is:
2) An essential part of nursing care

15: Adjuvant drugs are:
4) Used alongside analgesics

16: Non-pharmacological methods of pain control are:
1) Complementary to analgesics